Let's get Coffee

The History & Health Benefits of Coffee

Joe Urbach

www.gardeningaustin.com

www.phytonutrientfarms.com

A

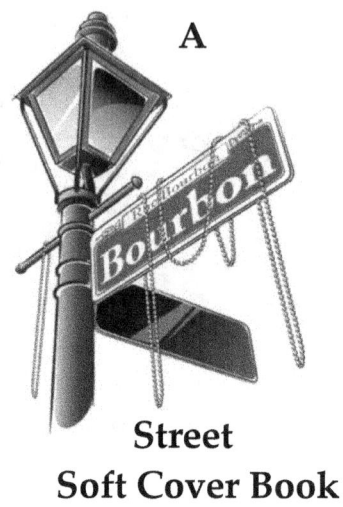

Street
Soft Cover Book

1st published in the United State in 2017 by
Bond Street Publications, a Hojo Enterprises Company

1st Printing 2017

Copyright © Joseph Urbach 2017

All rights reserved under International and Pan-American Copyright Conventions.

DEDICATION

For my Mother,
whose love of coffee peculates in me
and automatically drips down to my children!

"Let us raise our demitasse cups, our favorite old mugs, and our commuter cups to toast the thieves and smugglers to whom we truly owe our gratitude. These unsung and unsavory heroes set forth the proliferation of coffee throughout the world and the variety of species we cherish today.

Let us thank those who, through the centuries toiled, battled, tinkered and seduced, all for that delectable cup of coffee, and for all of those who brought us to this wonderful place in coffee history, this book is for you!"

CONTENTS

Forward

I am not a scientist, nor a medical doctor, nor a nutritionist nor any other kind of healthcare worker. I am not a research professional nor have I ever been involved in medical research of any kind.

I am a gardener, a father, a grandfather, and a diabetic. All of this led me to my concern about nutrition, and in turn, led me on a quest that eventually led to the writing of my **_Yes, Food IS Medicine_** series of books (originally titled 'Phytonutrient Gardening'). My journey of exploration has convinced me that There is a serious PROBLEM with the NUTRITION-LESS state of the modern fruits and vegetables that are

finding their way into our local markets and eventually on to our dinner plates. The real concern is that it soon can impact our health. In addition, half of the children on planet Earth live in poverty conditions, many suffering malnutrition and forced to drink polluted or tainted water. In this day and age, with all the modern advances of man, this situation is completely unacceptable and that is why I had to write that series.

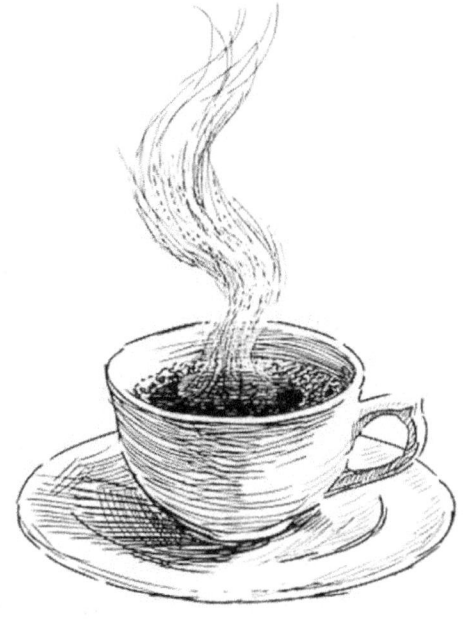

So, like many of you, I set off in search of helpful health information – but alas, most of what I found was of little merit and even less use. I found misinformation, false information and outright lies. Much of the worst of the 'garbage' info I found revolved around one of my favorite beverages – coffee. I knew that someone was going to have to set the record straight; so, why not me!

The information I present in this work is provided for your consideration only and I absolutely do not condone, endorse, or recommend that you suddenly take up drinking copious amounts of coffee in some crazy, misguided attempt to find a quick and easy health fix. No. I do not even suggest you change any of your diet or exercise habits without first consulting your healthcare professional.

My honest belief is that knowledge is power and my goal is to empower you with the information that follows so that you and your doctor can choose the best course of action for you to take to help you achieve a better, healthier, happier, and longer life!

I Am Not A Doctor

The information presented here is accurate to the best of my knowledge.

I am not a doctor therefore this information is not intended to diagnose, treat, cure or prevent any disease because only doctors can do that.

Please do your own research!

INTRODUCTION

I simply cannot start my day without a hot cup of coffee or two. The smell of a fresh pot of java percolating away is absolutely heaven. Nothing says, "Good Morning, Joe" like my first cup!

The more research I do into nutrition and how the food and drinks we consume relates to our health, the more I discover a simple truth that modern man has somehow gotten all screwed up. That simple truth is that the very thought of almost any food or drink being inherently bad for us is just plain hogwash! This is especially true when it comes to my morning java!

There are concerns, too much caffeine is certainly trouble, no one can deny that, but the solution to this concern is moderation. As is so often true in life, moderation is the key. Coffee and the caffeine that even decaffeinated coffee contains are not at all bad for us, and in fact, offer many health benefits when consumed in moderation! Let me say this again: **Moderation in our consumption and enjoyment of almost anything, as with so much in life, is key.**

But how much is considered moderate and how much is too much? How has coffee influenced mankind throughout history? Just what benefits does this 'Nectar of the Gods' have to offer us?

Those were the very questions I set out to answer as I sat at my computer one morning to write a post for my Phytonutrient Blog. I started researching and writing and before I knew it I was no longer writing a blog post but had just started my next book! The result is in your hands. I hope you enjoy reading it as much as I enjoyed writing it!

Chapter 1: Coffee is History

It may well surprise you to learn that there is no precise account of the origins of the coffee plant or of the first human consumption of the revered bean, though there is agreement among historians that coffee was first discovered in the mountains of Ethiopia (Abyssinia). Well, general agreement. Okay, at least basic agreement. No, the fact is that there is not much real agreement at all to be honest!

Google "Origins of Coffee" and you get more than 8 million results. More noteworthy than sheer numbers are the differing schools of thought that click-throughs reveal, right on page one. Depending on whom you trust, coffee was discovered around the 13th century. Or the fifth century. Or perhaps one of six other different periods in ancient times.

Coffee's history comprises yet another great debate, like preparation method and bean source; one more example of deeply felt passion for coffee on display. Such intellectual debate is entirely fitting for a beverage known to stir provocative thought. The coffeehouse's roots as a place for free idea exchange and political conversation in the 16th century Ottoman Empire are historically well established.

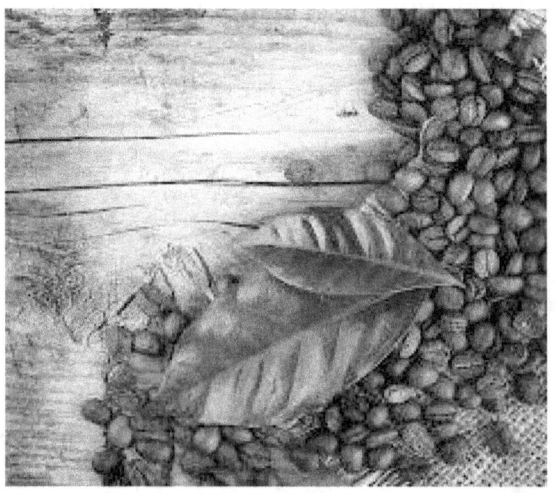

But I'm jumping ahead. Let me rewind, and start by asking a question that may at first seem fairly ridiculous…

What is coffee?

Everyone recognizes a roasted coffee bean, but you might not recognize an actual coffee plant with its berry covered branches. Did you know that coffee grows on trees? It does, though most people think the beans grow on a bush because coffee trees are pruned short to conserve their energy and to aid in harvesting, but they can grow to more than 30 feet high when left unpruned.

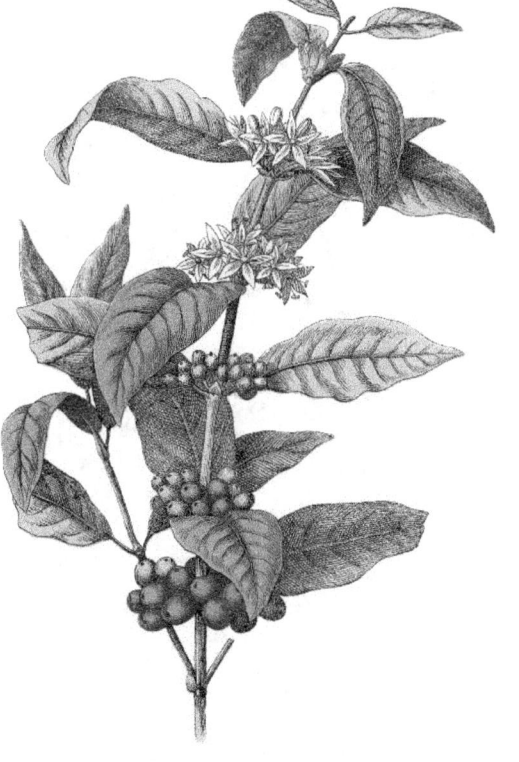

Each tree is covered with green, waxy leaves growing opposite each other in pairs. Coffee cherries grow along the branches. Because it grows in a continuous cycle, it's not unusual to see flowers, green fruit and ripe fruit simultaneously on a single tree.

It takes nearly a year for a cherry to mature after first flowering, and about 5 years of growth to reach full fruit production. While coffee plants can live up to 100 years, they are generally the most productive between the ages of 7 and 20. Proper care can maintain and even increase their output over the years, depending on the variety. The average coffee tree produces 10 pounds of coffee cherry per year, or 2 pounds of green beans.

All commercially grown coffee is from a region of the world called the Coffee Belt. The trees grow best in rich soil, with mild temperatures, frequent rain and shaded sun.

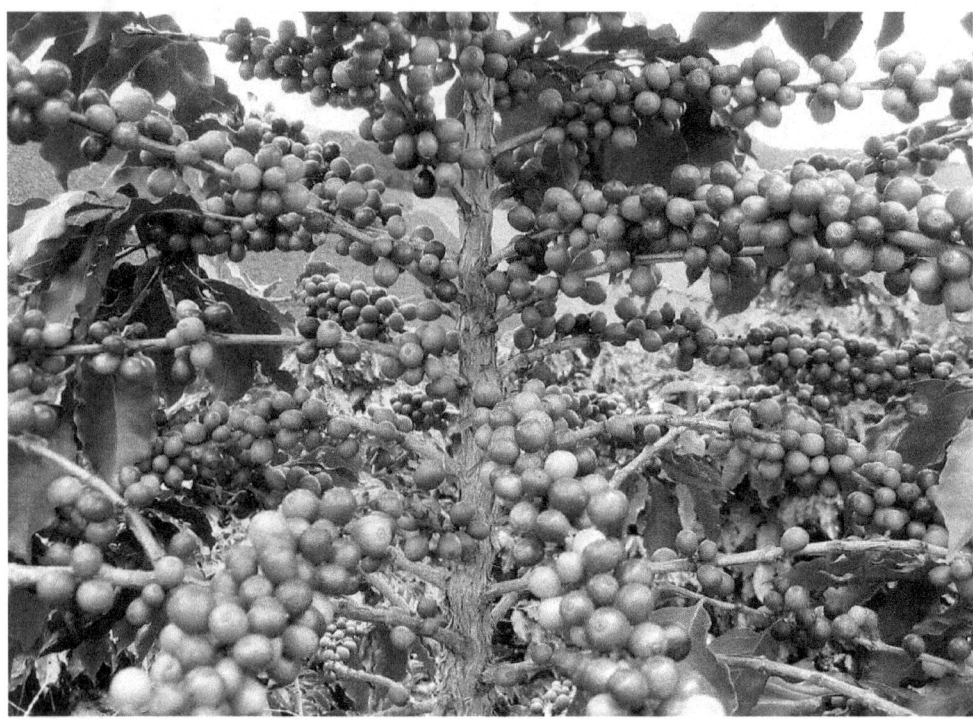

Coffee traces its origin to a genus of plants known as *Coffea*. Within the genus there are over 500 genera and 6,000 species of tropical trees and shrubs. Experts estimate that there are anywhere from 25 to 100 species of coffee plants.

The genus was first described in the 18th century by the Swedish botanist, Carolus Linneaus, who also described Coffea Arabica in his Species Plantarum in 1753. Botanists have disagreed ever since on the exact classification, since coffee plants can range widely. They can appear to be small shrubs or tall trees, with leaves from one to

16 inches in size, and in colors from purple or yellow to the predominant dark green.

In the commercial coffee industry, there are two important coffee species — Arabica and Robusta.

Coffea Arabica – Arabica is descended from the original coffee trees discovered in Ethiopia. These trees produce a fine, mild, aromatic coffee and represent approximately 70% of the world's coffee production. The beans are flatter and more elongated than Robusta and lower in caffeine.

On the world market, Arabica coffees bring the highest prices. The better Arabicas are high grown coffees — generally grown between 2,000 to 6,000 feet (610 to 1830 meters) above sea level — though optimal altitude varies with proximity to the equator. The most important factor is that temperatures must remain mild, ideally between 59 - 75 degrees Fahrenheit, with about 60 inches of rainfall a year. The trees are hearty, but a heavy frost will kill them. Arabica trees are costly to cultivate because the ideal terrain tends to be steep and access is difficult. Also, because the trees are more disease-prone than Robusta, they require additional care and attention.

Coffea Robusta - Most of the world's Robusta is grown in Central and Western Africa, parts of Southeast Asia, including Indonesia and Vietnam, and in Brazil. Production of Robusta is increasing, though it accounts for only about 30% of the world market.

Robusta is primarily used in blends and for instant coffees. The Robusta bean itself tends to be slightly rounder and smaller than an Arabica bean. The Robusta tree is heartier and more resistant to disease and parasites, which makes it easier and cheaper to cultivate.

It also has the advantage of being able to withstand warmer climates, preferring constant temperatures between 75 and 85 degrees Fahrenheit, which enables it to grow at far lower altitudes than Arabica. Still, it requires about 60 inches of rainfall a year, and cannot withstand frost. Compared with Arabica, Robusta beans produce a coffee which has a distinctive taste and about 50-60% more caffeine.

The beans you brew are actually the processed and roasted seeds from a fruit, which is called a coffee cherry. The coffee cherry's outer skin is called the *exocarp*. Beneath it is the *mesocarp*, a thin layer of pulp, followed by a slimy layer called the *parenchyma*. The beans themselves are covered in a paper-like envelope named the *exocarp*, more commonly referred to as *the parchment*.

Inside the parchment, side-by-side, lie two beans, each covered separately by yet another thin membrane. The biological name for this seed skin is the *spermoderm*, but it is generally referred to in the coffee trade as the *silver skin*.

In about 5% of the world's coffee, there is only one bean inside the cherry. This is called a peaberry (or a *caracol*, or "snail" in Spanish),

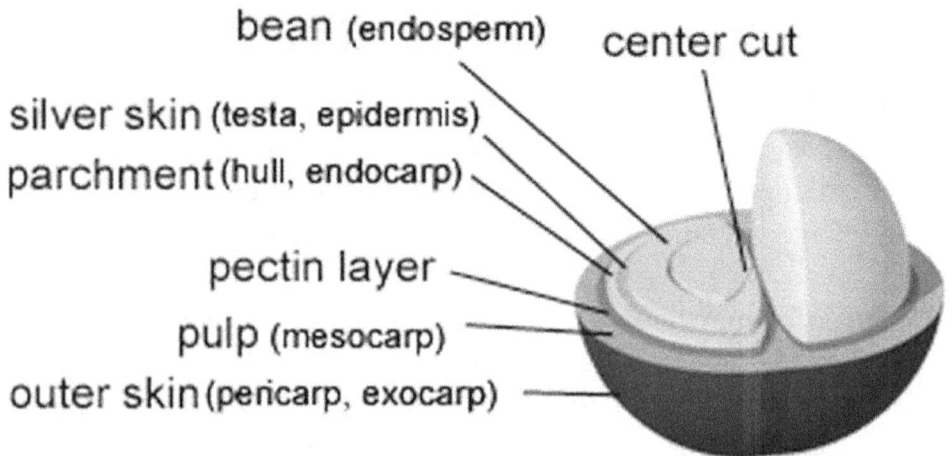

bean (endosperm)   center cut

silver skin (testa, epidermis)
parchment (hull, endocarp)

pectin layer
pulp (mesocarp)
outer skin (pericarp, exocarp)

and it is a natural mutation. Some people believe that peaberries are actually sweeter and more flavorful than standard beans, so they are sometimes manually sorted out for special sale.

Regardless of which variety of coffee bean your favorite 'cup of joe' is filled with, between the time they're planted, picked and purchased, any coffee beans go through a typical series of steps to bring out their best.

First off, the coffee tree has to be planted. A coffee bean is actually a seed. When dried, roasted and ground, it's used to brew coffee. If the seed isn't processed, but rather treated like any other seed, it can be planted and grow into a coffee tree.

Coffee seeds are generally planted in large beds in shaded nurseries. The seedlings will be watered frequently and shaded from bright sunlight until they are hearty enough to be permanently planted. Planting often takes place during the wet season, so that the soil remains moist while the roots become firmly established. Depending on the variety, weather, sun and many other variables, it will take approximately 3 to 5 years for the newly planted coffee trees to bear fruit.

The fruit, called the coffee cherry, turns a bright, deep red when it is ripe and ready to be harvested. There is typically one major harvest a year. In countries like Colombia, where there are two flowerings annually, there is a main crop and secondary, slightly smaller crop. In most countries, the crop is picked by hand in a labor-intensive and difficult process, though in places like Brazil where the landscape is relatively flat and the coffee fields are immense, the process has been mechanized. Whether by hand or by machine, all coffee is harvested in one of two ways:

- **Strip Picked**: All of the cherries are stripped off of the branch at one time, either by machine or by hand.
- **Selectively Picked:** Only the ripe cherries are harvested, and they are picked individually by hand. Pickers rotate among the trees every eight to 10 days, choosing only the cherries which are at the peak of ripeness. Because this kind of harvest is labor intensive and much more costly, it is used primarily to harvest the finer Arabica beans.

A good picker averages approximately 100 to 200 pounds of coffee cherries each day, which will produce 20 to 40 pounds of coffee beans. Each worker's daily haul is carefully weighed, and each picker is paid on the merit of his or her work. The day's harvest is then transported to the processing plant.

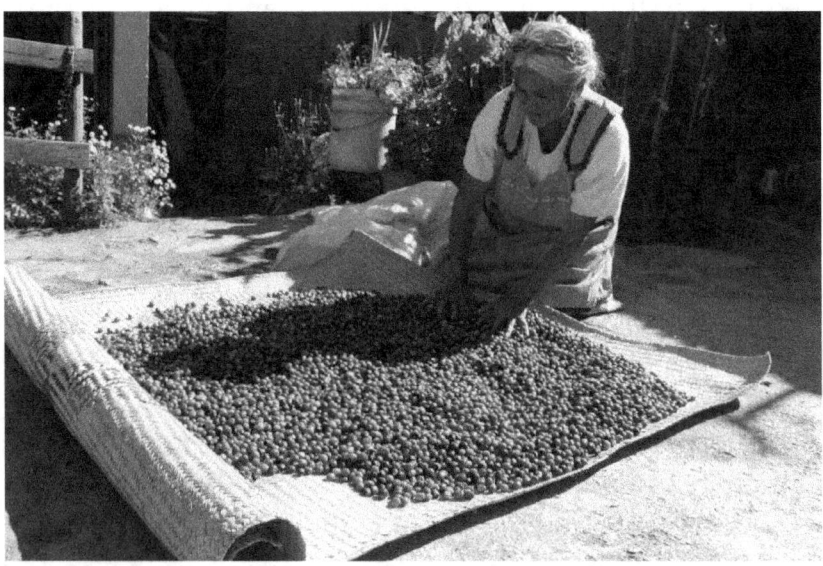

Once the coffee has been picked, processing must begin as quickly as possible to prevent fruit spoilage. Depending on location and local resources, coffee is processed in one of two ways:

- **The Dry Method** is the age-old method of processing coffee, and still used in many countries where water resources are limited. The freshly picked cherries are simply spread out on huge surfaces to dry in the sun. In order to prevent the cherries from spoiling, they are raked and turned throughout the day, then covered at night or during rain to prevent them from getting wet. Depending on the weather, this process might continue for several weeks for each batch of coffee until the moisture content of the cherries drops to 11%.
- **The Wet Method** removes the pulp from the coffee cherry after harvesting so the bean is dried with only the parchment skin left on. First, the freshly harvested cherries are passed through a pulping machine to separate the skin and pulp from the bean.

Then the beans are separated by weight as they pass through water channels. The lighter beans float to the top, while the heavier ripe beans sink to the bottom. They are passed through a series of rotating drums which separate them by size.

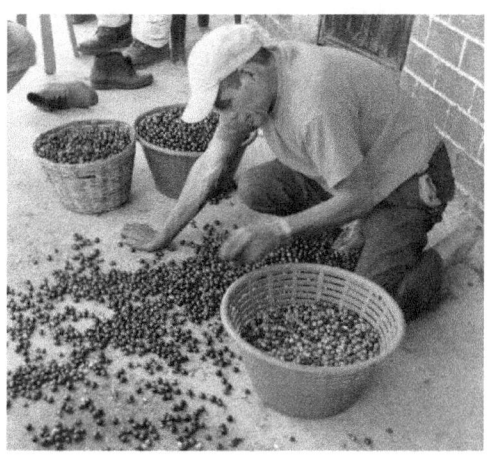

After separation, the beans are transported to large, water-filled fermentation tanks. Depending on a combination of factors -- such as the condition of the beans, the climate and even the altitude at which they are processed -- they will remain in these tanks for anywhere from 12 to 48 hours to remove the slick layer of mucilage (called the *parenchyma*) that is still attached to the parchment. While resting in the tanks, naturally occurring enzymes will cause this layer to dissolve.

When fermentation is complete, the beans feel rough to the touch. The beans are rinsed by going through additional water channels, and are ready for drying.

If the beans have been processed by the wet method, the pulped and fermented beans must now be dried to approximately 11% moisture to properly prepare them for storage. These beans, still inside the parchment envelope (the *endocarp*), can be sun-dried by spreading them on drying tables or floors, where they are turned regularly, or they can be machine-dried in large tumblers. The dried beans are known as *parchment coffee*, and are warehoused in jute or sisal bags until they are readied for export. Before being exported, *parchment coffee* is processed in the following manner:

- **Hulling** machinery removes the parchment layer (*endocarp*) from wet processed coffee. Hulling dry processed coffee refers to removing the entire dried husk — the *exocarp, mesocarp* and *endocarp* — of the dried cherries.
- **Polishing** is an optional process where any silver skin that remains on the beans after hulling is removed by machine. While polished beans are considered superior to unpolished ones, in reality, there is little difference between the two.
- **Grading and Sorting** is done by size and weight, and beans are also reviewed for color flaws or other imperfections.

Beans are sized by being passed through a series of screens. They are also sorted pneumatically by using an air jet to separate heavy from light beans.

Typically, the bean size is represented on a scale of 10 to 20. The number represents the size of a round hole's diameter in terms of 1/64's of an inch. A number 10 bean would be the approximate size of a hole in a diameter of 10/64 of an inch, and a number 15 bean, 15/64 of an inch. I have no idea who came up with this system but it is used industry wide.

Finally, defective beans are removed either by hand or by machinery. Beans that are unsatisfactory due to deficiencies (unacceptable size or color, over-fermented beans, insect-damaged, unhulled, etc.) are removed. In many countries, this process is done both by machine and by hand, ensuring that only the finest quality coffee beans are exported.

The milled beans, now referred to as *green coffee*, are loaded onto ships in either jute or sisal bags loaded in shipping containers, or bulk-shipped inside plastic-lined containers. World coffee production for 2015/16 was 152.7 million 60-kg bags, according to information provided by the USDA Foreign Agriculture Service. Once shipped to the coffee distributors the journey isn't finished yet. You see, up to this point the coffee has not even been tasted!

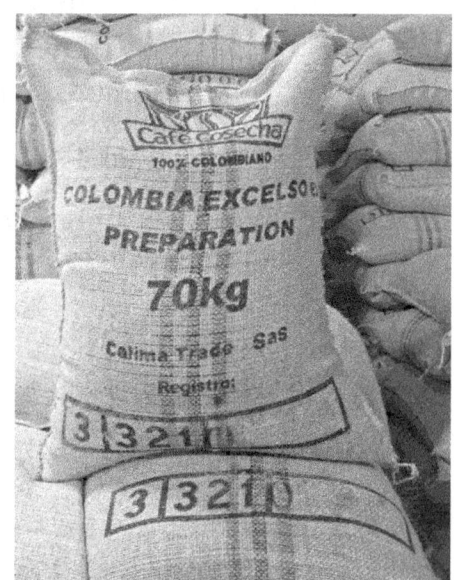

From this point on, the coffee is repeatedly tested for quality and taste. This process is referred to as *cupping* and usually takes place in a room specifically designed to facilitate the process.

- First, the taster — usually called the *cupper* — evaluates the beans for their overall visual quality. The beans are then roasted in a small laboratory roaster, immediately ground and infused in boiling water with carefully-controlled temperature. The cupper *noses* the brew to experience its aroma, an essential step in judging the coffee's quality.
- After letting the coffee rest for several minutes, the cupper breaks the crust by pushing aside the grounds at the top of the cup. Again, the coffee is *nosed* before the tasting begins.
- To taste the coffee, the cupper slurps a spoonful with a quick inhalation. The objective is to spray the coffee evenly over the cupper's taste buds, and then weigh it on the tongue before spitting it out.

Samples from a variety of batches and different beans are tasted daily. Coffees are not only analyzed to determine their flaws and characteristics, but also for the purpose of blending different beans or creating the proper roast. An expert cupper can taste hundreds of samples of coffee a day and still taste the subtle differences between them. Much like those professional wine experts, I find this ability simple amazing.

Finally, it is time to roast the coffee beans. Roasting transforms green coffee into the aromatic brown beans that we purchase in our favorite stores or cafés. Most roasting machines maintain a temperature of about 550 degrees Fahrenheit. The beans are kept moving throughout the entire process to keep them from burning.

When they reach an internal temperature of about 400 degrees Fahrenheit, they begin to turn brown and the *caffeol*, a fragrant oil locked inside the beans, begins to emerge. This process called *pyrolysis* is at the heart of roasting — it produces the flavor and aroma of the coffee we drink.

After roasting, the beans are immediately cooled either by air or water. Roasting is generally performed in the importing countries because freshly roasted beans must reach the consumer as quickly as possible.

At this point, we are just about ready to brew our morning cup, first though, we need to grind the beans. The objective of a proper grind is to get the most flavor in a cup of coffee. How coarse or fine the coffee is ground depends on the brewing method. The length of time the grounds will be in contact with water determines the ideal grade of grind Generally, the finer the grind, the more quickly the coffee should be prepared. That's why coffee ground for an espresso machine is much finer than coffee brewed in a drip system.

Should you make your coffee from whole bean that you grind just before you brew your pot or should you purchase pre-ground coffee beans? That is the question, and it can be quite the debate among coffee connoisseurs, with both sides of the story having some positives and negatives. Most people buy and use ground coffee, mainly because that is the easiest to use and the form that is found on the shelves of every local supermarket. It's ready to brew, and won't require any extra time, skills or equipment on your part. And that pretty much sums up all the positive aspects of pre-ground coffee. Ease and convenience.

People also lean towards ground coffee because they wouldn't know what to do with whole bean coffee. There are a few pitfalls to ground coffee though, so you might want to think twice about taking that route. The most important one is freshness. Once it's been roasted and ground, coffee will go stale fast. All the taste is in the bean oils, and they will evaporate once the beans are ground up. Even cans of coffee that have been vacuum-packed are going to be much less fresh than coffee you grind yourself. If you've never had freshly ground coffee, you may not even realize there is a difference. But take my word for it, there is quite a difference!

If you buy whole beans, and then grind them up minutes before you brew up your pot of coffee, the flavor is much stronger and the subtle tastes of your specific type of bean are more noticeable. The second thing to consider when comparing whole bean to ground coffee is grind fineness. Depending on what brand of ground coffee you buy, you usually don't get to select how fine or coarse you want. Different brewing methods work best with different types of coarseness, so why limit yourself to only one option? If you grind it yourself, you can make up a batch of coarse coffee for your French press or some fine grinds for an espresso machine Even the simplest coffee bean grinder will give you the control over your grounds. Since you'll only be grinding small amounts right before you brew, you can change the fineness whenever you want.

So, even with these issues between whole bean and ground coffee, there is still the problem of the extra effort involved in doing the grinding yourself. That would be the main downfall for whole beans. In truth, it only takes a minute or two to grind up enough beans for a pot of coffee so the effort is minimal once you get into the habit of doing it.

Cleaning out the coffee grinder can also be a bit of a chore. And the grinder itself is another downside to whole bean coffee. Not everyone wants another piece of kitchen equipment around. You can buy small and inexpensive models, or spend quite a bit more on a grinder with more controls and features. A burr grinder will produce the most even grind, but blade grinders are much cheaper. The bottom line is that between whole bean and ground coffee, the things to consider are freshness, control and convenience. Whole beans will give you a fresher cup and you can decide your own level of coarseness, but ground coffee is ready without any work.

For those of us who make coffee an important part of their life another option is available, use both whole and ground! When I am pressed for time or just feeling lazy I opt for the ground coffee. But on cold Sunday morning when I have no time constraints nothing beats fresh grinding whole beans to make the perfect cup of coffee.

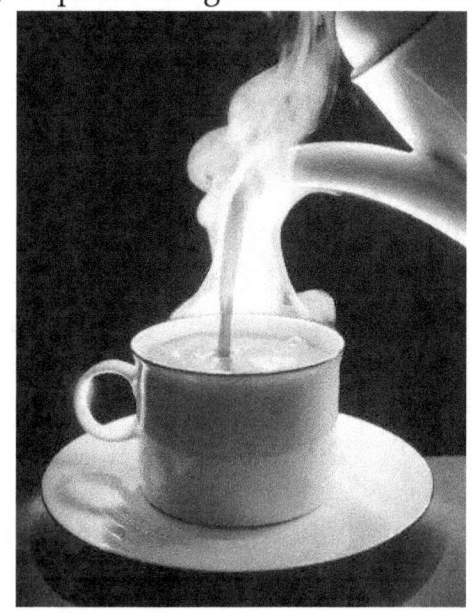

Now, finally, I have our cup of coffee, I can sit back and enjoy! I am doing just that right now and there may be no better way to spend a small chunk of your day than how I am right now. Relaxing with a hot cup of coffee and watching my wife play with our grandson on the floor of the living room. Life can be really good!

Chapter 2: The Early Years

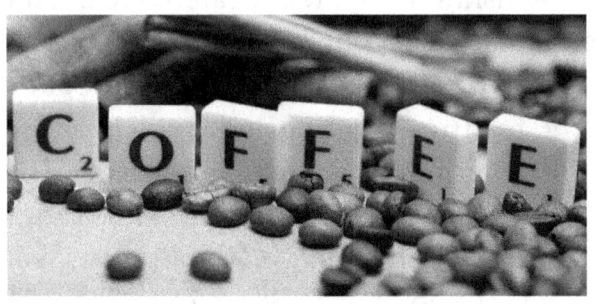

The history of coffee... a simple timeline of events? I think not! No, the journey of coffee, my friends, is so much more. It's a swashbuckling adventure spanning a thousand years, filled with death-defying escapes, international intrigue and - oh yes! - torrid romance. From distant, tropical islands to the power centers of international trade, it has been banned, berated, hailed and championed, generating as much fear as enjoyment. This is not just a drink, this is magic, infusing itself into our psyche, stirring conflict and controversy. Read on, friends, and enjoy the bold, robust voyage that is coffee.

According to a coffee history legend, an Arabian shepherd named Kaldi found his goats dancing joyously around a dark green leafed shrub with bright red cherries in the southern tip of the Arabian Peninsula. Kaldi soon determined that it was the bright red cherries on the shrub that were causing the peculiar euphoria and after trying the cherries himself, he learned of their powerful effect.

Kaldi reported his findings to the abbot of the local monastery, "These berries are heaven sent." At first the abbot, was underwhelmed, "Are you possessed?" He condemned the berries as the Devil's work and promptly threw them into the fire. "Evil!"

But soon after, the smell of fresh roasted coffee filled the pious halls of the monastery, enticing the monks. After the chief monk dozed off, (due to the lack of caffeine mind you,) a young rebellious monk snatched the cooling beans from the fire pit. This innovator, the world's first barista, mixed the beans with water and the resulting brew kept the monks up all night thanking their creator. "Hallelujah!" Quite a holy revelation, indeed!

Meanwhile, word of these fragrant, energizing berries traveled to another corner of Ethiopia and caught the imagination of the Galla tribe. The Galla mixed the berry with ghee, a clarified butter, and pressed the mixture into a scrumptious power bar. Their warriors marched into battle with their new, energizing snack and were invincible! In fact, similar bars are still eaten in Kaffa and Sidamo, Ethiopia to this day.

Another traditional legend about the first discovery of coffee involves an Arabian mystic named Omar who was exiled to the desert by his enemies. Omar faced imminent starvation until he made a broth from the berries of coffee trees and was able to stay alive. Residents of the nearby town of Mocha thought Omar's survival was a religious sign.

The Mocha region continues to be a major coffee source today. Mocha is also well known as the place where the first coffee beans that became popular in Europe were produced.

Despite the appeal of such legends, recent botanical evidence suggests a different coffee bean origin. This evidence indicates that the history of the coffee bean began on the plateaus of central Ethiopia and somehow must have been brought to Yemen where it was cultivated since the 6th century. Upon introduction of the first coffee houses in Cairo and Mecca coffee became a passion rather than just a stimulant.

We do know for sure that the coffee plant originated from a plateau in Ethiopia, given its proclivity for spontaneous growth there as nowhere else. The region is known as Kaffa. It's not clear if coffee took its name from the region, or vice versa. So, it's a short leap to assume that coffee was first consumed on a large scale in Ethiopia, and to figure out roughly when. Well, not so easy, and not so fast. We can't know either for sure.

There is no documentation, so I came up my own theory. I imagine one of our starved ancestors (thousands or millions of years ago) walking around what is now Ethiopia looking for something to eat. Desperate, ravenous, he discovers a bush full of red fruit. He's a little worried. He doesn't know if it's poisonous, but left with little choice, he picks a cherry and puts it in his month. He finds a relatively un-pulpy inside, along with two big beans.

The taste is sweet, signaling nourishment. *"Maybe this is okay,"* he thinks. He continues eating until he feels satiated, and realizes he feels more than just full. He feels rested, awake; his reflexes are alive. When night comes, he can't sleep. He likes this sensation—all these sensations—and decides to bring this new fruits to his people. And quite possibly from that moment, coffee (if not yet its beverage form) becomes part of his tribe's diet.

The earliest records of coffee in history, that archaeologists can confirm, teaches us that, at first, coffee was not used as a drink, between 575 and 850 A.D. it was used as a food. The coffee beans were crushed into balls mixed with animal fat and eaten as quick, rough-hewn, high energy snacks that were used to invigorate weary

Ethiopian travellers and hard marching warriors. The fat, protein and caffeine in the balls provided energy and alertness, making an early form of energy bar!

Coffee first begin to be made into a drink around 1000 A.D. and was first written about at that time, by physician and philosopher Avicenna of Bukhara. Abu 'Ali al-Husayn ibn Sina, better known in Europe by the Latinized name "Avicenna" was the most significant philosopher in the Islamic tradition and arguably the most influential philosopher of the pre-modern era. Born in Afshana near Bukhara in Central Asia in about 980, he was best known as a polymath, as a physician whose major work the *Canon (al-Qanun fi'l-Tibb)* continued to be taught as a medical textbook in Europe and in the Islamic world until the early modern period, and as a philosopher whose major *summa* the *Cure (al-Shifa')* had a decisive impact upon European scholasticism.

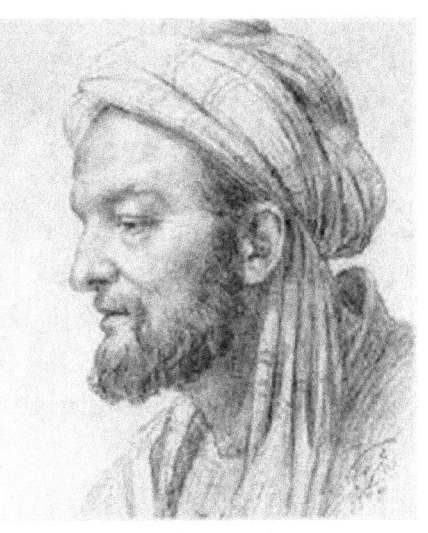

Avicenna wrote, *"It fortifies the members, it cleans the skin, and dries up the humidities that are under it and gives an excellent smell to all the body."*

Early writings establish Yemen, on the southern part of the Arabian Peninsula, just across the Red Sea from Ethiopia, as home to the first coffee plantations, starting in the early 15th century. Coffee plants were brought over from Ethiopia, Yemen lacking its own indigenous coffee. There, Sufi monks prepared an infusion of coffee cherry leaves to stay awake and pray through the night. The first real roasting and grinding activities likely happened here.

Coffee's true worldwide journey came with the Turkish conquests of the Arabian Peninsula, it was the Ottoman Empire that brought coffee to entirely new places, for new reasons.

The Muslim religion's prohibition of alcohol consumption gave a big lift to coffee throughout Turkey and the rest of the Ottoman Empire. Coffee became a substitute for wine, and was given the name *kahve* — literally, "wine of Arabia." The word came from the Arabic term *oahwah*, itself from the verb *oahiya*, signifying the action of feeling sated.

Coffee diffused quickly throughout the Ottoman Empire. By the 1100's enterprising Arab traders return to their homeland, now modern-day Yemen, with coffee from Ethiopia. They cultivate the plant for the first time on plantations and create a most satisfying, uplifting drink by boiling the beans in water. It was called "qahwa" meaning *"that which prevents sleep."*

Incidentally, qahwa, also written as "kahwah", is one of many words Arabs used for wine. You see, in the process of stripping the coffee bean's cherry-like husk, the pulp could then be fermented to make a potent, alcoholic beverage with quite a kick in the palate!

The bottom line for coffee's ancient history is simply this, those who consumed it early on were after the stimulant substance it contained, that alkaloid well known today as caffeine. All of coffee's legends tell of its energizing effect, from Kaldi's goats to Mahomet, who, after consuming a hot, black liquid given to him by the angel Gabriel, promptly removed 40 knights from their horses, and satisfied 40 virgins in just one day. (Take that, Viagra!)

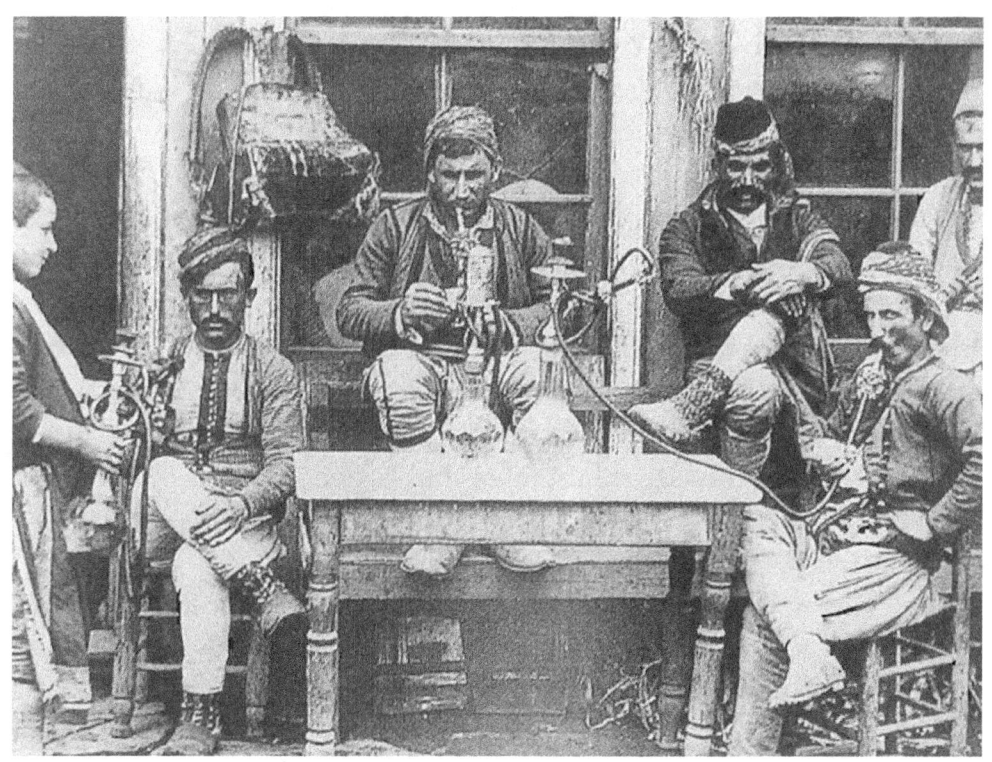

Come the early 1400's Ottoman Turks introduced coffee to the bustling power center of Constantinople. Those clever Turks added clove, cardamom, cinnamon and anise to their brew and created a most spicy, energizing concoction. If you ever find yourself in Istanbul, order this blast from the past that is still enjoyed to this day.

In 1454, The Mufti of Aden visited the Ethiopian countryside and saw his own citizens drinking coffee. He demanded that he be given a taste! The drink, it was written, *"cures him of some unknown affliction."* Naturally, he approved of the drink straight away. His approval helped spread coffee's popularity all the way to Mecca.

So, we now know that coffee cultivation and trade began on the Arabian Peninsula. By the 15th century, coffee was being grown in the Yemeni district of Arabia and by the 16th century it was known in Persia, Egypt, Syria, and Turkey.

Coffee shops were soon opening in Constantinople around this same time, which many claim were the first 'modern' coffee houses. They quickly became hotspots for lively discussions and political debates. In fact, coffee became so much a part of Turkish culture that they create a law that made it legal for a woman to divorce her husband if he failed to provide her with her daily quota of coffee beans. Some believe that this was where the idea that coffee is an aphrodisiac got its start.

Coffee was not only enjoyed in homes, but also in the many public coffee houses — called *qahveh khaneh* — which began to appear in cities across the Near East. The popularity of the coffee houses was unequaled and people frequented them for all kinds of social activity.

Not only did the patrons drink coffee and engage in conversation, but they also listened to music, watched performers, played chess and kept current on the news. Coffee houses quickly became such an important center for the exchange of information that they were often referred to as "Schools of the Wise."

With thousands of pilgrims visiting the holy city of Mecca each year from all over the world, knowledge of this "wine of Araby" began to spread.

Chapter 3: Coffee Hits Europe

At this point, Arabia and Muslim Africa enjoyed a monopoly on coffee production; In order to keep it that way, their laws forbid the export of fertile beans. Fertile beans are those with the cherry still around the seed. Before they were exported, coffee beans were boiled to make them infertile by shedding the husk off to prevent clever smugglers from sneaking away with the precious goods. But nothing is fool-proof...

After his pilgrimage to Mecca, an Asian Indian named Baba Budan manages to leave the Muslim city with a few fertile coffee beans concealed against his stomach. After returning to India, he secretly cultivates the beans. The descendants of those well-traveled beans are still producing coffee to this day! In fact, "Old Chik", as the original beans are known, account for approximately a third of the coffee India produces. No wonder Baba Budan was made a Saint and there's a region of India named after him.

European travelers to India and the Near East brought back stories of an unusual dark black beverage. The early 17th century saw Muslim coffee's introduction to Christian Europe, through the work of Venetian merchants and in no time coffee was becoming popular across the continent.

Some people reacted to this new beverage with suspicion or fear, it met with strong resistance from the Catholic Church, especially by the Pope's Councilmen, who asked Pope Clemente VIII to declare the black beverage "the bitter invention of Satan." This 'great controversy' grew so fast and caused such a stir, that Pope Clement

VIII finally decided to intervene. Before he would rule on the drink, however, he opted to taste the dark liquid for himself. Fortunately for us all, he found the drink so satisfying that he gave it papal approval. In fact, he liked what he tasted so much that he is said to have declared, "this devil's drink is so delicious... we should cheat the devil by baptizing it!"

Despite such controversy, coffee houses were quickly becoming centers of social activity and communication in the major cities of England, Austria, France, Germany and Holland, just as they had in Arabia. In England, "penny universities" sprang up, so called because for the price of a penny, one could purchase a cup of coffee and engage in stimulating conversation.

Coffee began to replace the common breakfast drink beverages of the time — beer and wine. Those who drank coffee instead of alcohol began the day alert and energized, and not surprisingly, the quality of their work was greatly improved. (I like to think of this a precursor to the modern office coffee service.)

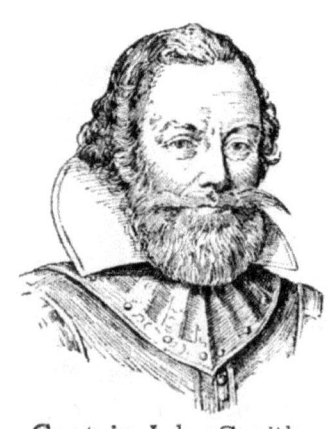

Captain John Smith.

The knowledge of coffee was making its way to the rest of the world. As early as 1607, Captain John Smith, a British world adventurer, who was one of the founders of the first English settlement Colony in Jamestown, Virginia, is known to have brought awareness of coffee to the newly discovered Americas. If fact, there's mention of the Turkish drink known as coffa in his bestselling book of the day _"Travels and Adventure."_ Perhaps it is a good cup of coffee that drove him to such amazing discoveries, dangerous adventures and into so much trouble too. Not only was the rabble-rouser nearly executed just as he arrived in the New World by his fellow Englishmen, he got into a tussle with the Natives as well.

Legend has it that while up-river, searching for food; he crossed the line and was captured by the Powhatan Tribe. Just before his execution, the Chief's beautiful 14 year-old daughter, Princess Pocahontas intervened. To spare him, she threw herself on top of the cocky Captain, willing to take a beating by clubs to protect him. The Chief relented to his daughter's compassion and apparently, her "school-girl" crush. Smith was freed. After the handsome and grateful Captain had spent some time with the young girl he set-off again. With a tip of his hat, a thank you and a wink, he left the brave young Princess Pocahontas behind. Rumor has it that these two had several rendezvous' over the next several years. Although some say that she was in love, I think she was in it for the coffee!

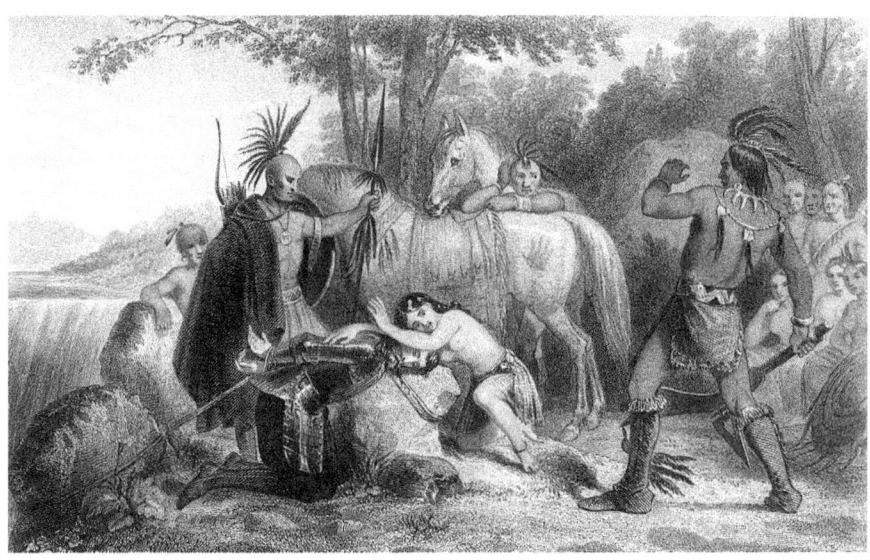

As early as the 1640s Europeans were starting to see that growing coffee might well prove a way to grow their fortunes. Successful cloth merchant and trader, Pieter Van Dan Broeck, was one of the first Dutchmen to taste coffee. While in the service of the Dutch East India Company, he visited Mocha in Yemen and drank "something hot and black." Since it was illegal to take a precious coffee plant or its fertile seeds/beans out of the Arab lands, Pieter set out to smuggle one back to the Netherlands. Unfortunately for the Dutch, and fortunate for the Yemenis, the cultivation in Holland fails miserably. Thwarted in Antwerp by the fickle little plant, that preferred the warmer temperatures of the equatorial zones, the Dutch soon discovered they couldn't grow this plant away from its origins as they had hoped. Not to be dissuaded, being the good businessmen they were, they set their sights on expanding from their near monopoly of the spice trade into coffee. They could see its potential and bided their time as they waited for the demand for coffee to take hold in Europe.

Also, around 1640, a Greek student at Oxford University brewed the very first cup of coffee in England. With his newfound get-up-and-go drink, Nathaniel Conopios would stay up all night throwing dishes and dancing, as well as cramming for those tricky tests, however Oxford's porcelain was more precious to them, than was young Nathaniel. He was summarily expelled. Back to Greece for poor him, yet coffee was in England to stay. It played an on-going role at energized Oxford University. Scientific breakthroughs were soon to come.

A few short years later the first coffee house in all of England opened near the University where eager students drove the drink's popularity. A few years after that, those caffeinated young men establish the 'Oxford Coffee Club'. None of those brainiacs were

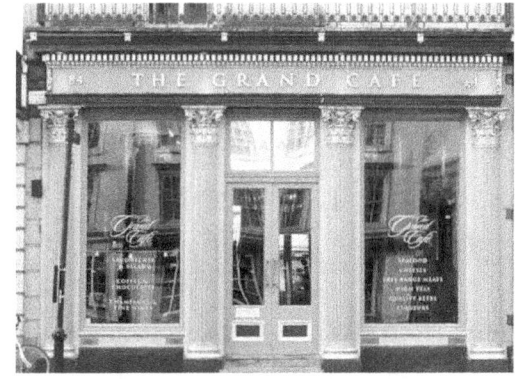

summarily expelled; instead the college all-nighter was born! -- And with it the creation of innovative theories and ideas shared not only by students, but also by leading scientists like Sir Robert Boyle. Years later the club would become the Royal Society, England's famous and respected world-renowned scientific think-tank. This building is now known as "The Grand Cafe." A plaque on the wall commemorates this and the Cafe is now a trendy cocktail bar.

Coffee's diffusion throughout Europe went at breakneck pace. Venice's first coffee house (*"bottega del caffe`"*) opened in 1645, England's in 1650, France's in 1672, In the mid-1600's, coffee was then brought to the New World, first in the town of New Amsterdam, later to be called New York by the British. A Boston coffee shop is known to have opened in 1676. Today's rapid proliferation of coffee houses? Well, it is nothing new, save perhaps for the free Wi-Fi.

Though coffee houses rapidly began to appear, tea continued to be the favored drink in the New World until 1773, when the colonists revolted against a heavy tax on tea imposed by King George III. The revolt, known as the Boston Tea Party, would forever change the American drinking preference to coffee, and by the way eventually led to a little conflict we have come to call the American Revolution.

By the mid-17th century, there were over 300 coffee houses in London, many of which attracted like-minded patrons, including merchants, shippers, brokers and artists.

A little-known factoid for you: In the late 1600s coffee overtook beer as New York City's favorite breakfast beverage - and it went much better with eggs, too!

Over in London, public drunkenness was a problem and coffee houses replaced taverns as the place of choice for meetings. Not wanting to see their profits shrink, tavern owners retaliated; they attacked the Arabic origins of coffee claiming it was not suitable for well-mannered Christian men, whereas Monks' have brewed beer for centuries. Many businesses grew out of these specialized coffee houses. Proprietor Edward Lloyd opened a coffee house in London. Lloyd mingled with his customers and created a list of their ships, the cargo they're carrying and the schedules they kept. Underwriters then use the list to sell insurance to those in need. Merchants tracked their ships and shipments. In time, Lloyd's of London became the world's best-known insurance company.

Oh, and incidentally... around this same time, the custom of tipping was born in English coffee houses. Customers place coins in a box labeled: "To Insure Prompt Service." T-I-P-S.

In the 1670s, an entrepreneurial Armenian named Pascal, first sold coffee to the Parisian public, he brewed it in a tent at the St. Germain spring fair. To increase sales, guided by his entrepreneurial spirit, Pascal sent his Turkish waiter boys throughout the streets of Paris, merrily yelling "Café! Café!" With pitcher and cups in hand, they pour and sell the steaming beverage door-to-door.

Coffee in Paris underwent a bit of a class war. The first evolution of coffee shops appealed mostly to the lower classes; the Paris elite avoided them. But before long more lavish shops opened with elegant, expensive décor. Tea and chocolates were offered in addition to coffee. Soon, the well-heeled men and fashionable women of Paris found themselves in attendance as Coffee was suddenly "en vogue."

As demand for the beverage continued to spread, there was fierce competition to cultivate coffee outside of Arabia. These beans quickly became precious and coffee plants much sought after. Big European empires like Holland and France tried to grow coffee in their own territories, far from the tropical climates where it was already known to best thrive. (Virtually all of the coffee we drink today is produced in regions situated in the tropics.) To preserve their monopoly, Arabian coffee traders intentionally made export beans infertile by parching or boiling them before export to Europe. The Dutch persevered, obtaining coffee plants and creating the first successful coffee plantation away from the Middle East, on their colony of Java in early 18th century Indonesia. They started with just a few coffee plants obtained through trade with merchants in the Yemenite port of Mocha. Mocha Java was born, its first shipment to Europe dating to 1719.

Following Java's success, coffee production was fast established on Sumatra and Ceylon. Some plants were cultivated in specially created botanical gardens in Amsterdam. As part of a military agreement, France received some of these plants as gifts in 1720, promptly transporting them to its colonies in Central America. A captain of the French Navy, Gabriel de Clieu, was ordered by King Louis XV to establish a plantation in Martinique. As the story goes, during the voyage, water was rationed, and the captain took care to share his portion with the plants. Recent findings points to coffee already growing in the French colony of Saint-Domingue as early as 1715, and in the Dutch colony of Surinam since 1718. So, the Dutch finally achieved success with their seedlings in the latter half of the

17th century. Their first attempts to plant them in India failed, but they were successful with their efforts in Batavia, on the island of Java in what is now Indonesia.

The plants thrived and soon the Dutch had a productive and growing trade in coffee. They then expanded the cultivation of coffee trees to the islands of Sumatra and Celebes.

The New World's tropical regions revealed themselves as ideal for cultivation, and coffee plantations spread throughout Central and South America. Central America's first coffee harvest occurred in 1726. Today, Brazil reigns as the world's biggest producer, claiming no fewer than 10 billion (billion, with a "b") coffee plants.

In 1675, in London, coffee was at the center in a war between the sexes. Women, you see, were barred from most male gatherings. So, if their men weren't at work or the pub, they were spending time at coffee houses - everywhere and anywhere but home. In fact, women surmised that coffee encouraged their men to drink more liquor. Hell hath no fury! So women circulate a petition entitled, "The Women's Petition against Coffee," which stated that coffee made their men impotent and was creating a "very sensible decay of that true Old English vigor." The men of England shot back, as men are apt to do, with "The Men's Answer to the Women's Petition against Coffee" claiming quite bluntly that coffee made their erections "more vigorous," the Ejaculation more full." Wow, the things people used to talk about!

Around this same time, though thoroughly unrelated to the lascivious claims of the warring sexes, King Charles II ordered England's coffee houses closed. Charles, it seems, is afraid of a war of a different kind: revolt. Coffee houses breed the kind of talk and ideas that might run counter to his royal rule.

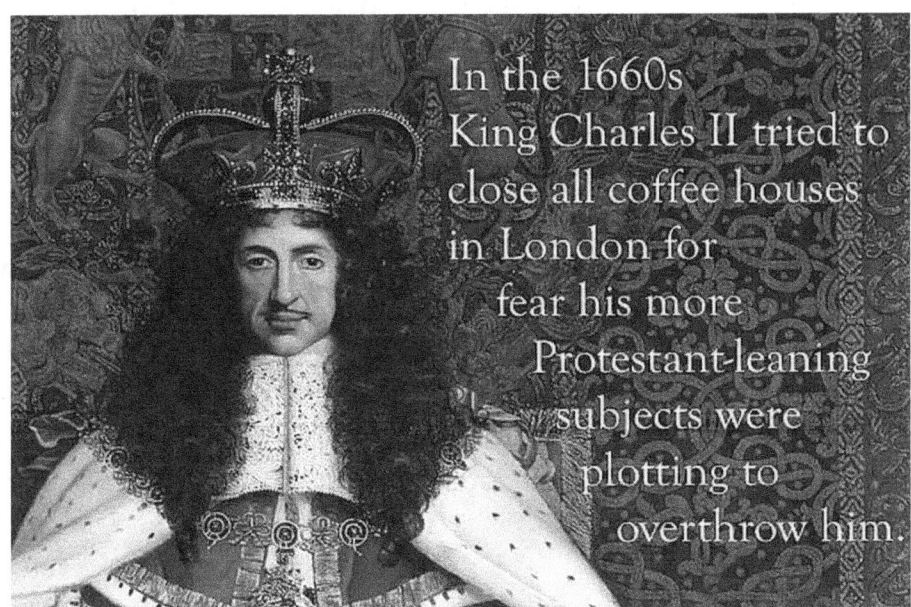

In the 1660s King Charles II tried to close all coffee houses in London for fear his more Protestant-leaning subjects were plotting to overthrow him.

A PROCLAMATION FOR THE SUPPRESSION OF COFFEE HOUSES:

"Whereas it is most apparent that the multitude of Coffee Houses of late years set up and kept within this Kingdom…and the great resort of idle and disaffected persons to them, have produced very much of their time, which might and probably would be employed in and about their Lawful Calling and Affairs; but also for that in such houses…divers, false, malitious, and scandalous reports are devised and spread abroad to the Defamation of His Majesty's Government, and to the disturbance of the Peace and Quiet of the Realm; his Majesty hath though it fit and necessary, that the said Coffee Houses be (for the Future) put down and suppressed…"

- King Charles II of England, December 23, 1675. This rule was revoked on January 8, just eleven days later, due to widespread citizen protest. Power to the people!

Here's a story of intrigue and heroism, in which a man on a secret mission and coffee were never the same thereafter. In 1683 the unstoppable Turkish Army of 300,000 laid siege and surrounded the Austrian city of Vienna for the second time. The grand city of culture was at the point of surrendering to the Ottoman Empire once and for all, even though help from an army of 33,000 Austrians was nearby. Odds did not favor the Viennese.

A man named Franz Georg Kolschitzky, a young Pole, who had lived in Istanbul for ten years and spoke Turkish, offered up his service to the beleaguered Viennese. Dressed in disguise, in the uniform of the Turkish Army, he clandestinely slipped through the enemy's lines. He gathered vital and strategic information. With this, the Prince of Lorraine and the Austrians attacked. The Turks fled, running so fast, they left their 25,000 tents, 10,000 Oxen, 5000 camels, and a tremendous bounty of Gold behind for the victors, yet to Franz, the true treasure abandoned was - 500 sacks of green coffee beans. The spoils were distributed; but no one wanted these odd little beans or knew what to do with them - except Franz, that is.

Franz was a hero! He was awarded Austrian nationality and granted permission to open the first Viennese coffee house... He named it the Blue Bottle. He made the coffee as he had learned in Istanbul. Most Viennese did not take to this strange new beverage. He brilliantly decided to filter the coffee, add a spoonful of cream and honey. Yummy! Business took off and he is known to this day as the Patron Saint to coffee houses in all of Vienna. Next time you order a Viennese Coffee, be sure to offer up a bit of thanks to one heroic young man versus 300,000 invaders and his reward of 500 sacks of beans!

The Italian Francesco Procopio dei Coltelli opened the Café Procope in Paris, in 1686. It has become known as the first literary coffee shop in the City of Lights. Patrons included Voltaire, whose table is still there, and the young lieutenant Napoleon Bonaparte, who once left his hat behind to settle his bill. Although Napoleon's hat is long gone, Café Procope is the oldest café in Paris and is still open today. It's located on the left bank at 13 rue de l'Ancienne Comédie.

Things really began to get moving now. The year was 1698 and something was brewing in London within Johnathan's Coffee House in Change Alley. John Castaing began to issue a list of stock and commodity prices. It is the earliest evidence of organized trading in marketable securities in London. Men gathered not only for their morning cup of coffee but to trade information and ended-up dealing in commodities. Alas, the London Stock Exchange was born, one of the world's oldest!

Time for a little more coffee intrigue... The Dutch did an odd thing that would eventually lead to the greatest heist in history! In 1714, the Mayor of Amsterdam presented a gift of a young coffee plant to King Louis XIV of France. The King ordered this most valuable of plant, be planted in the Royal Botanical Garden in Paris. Within the walled protection of the Royal Botanical Gardens it was on display for 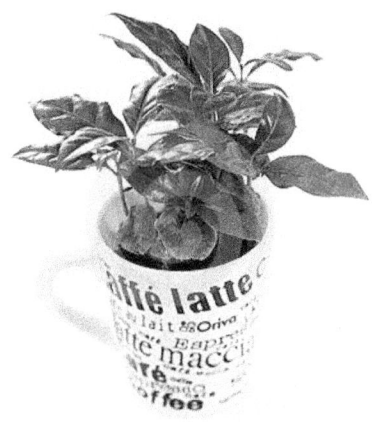 those in his court to be in awe of. He too would stop by and admire this singular coffee plant that could - that would... change the world.

Ten years would pass without incident, all was well in the Royal Botanical Garden. The coffee tree grew well and was the center of Garden and a favorite of the court. Yes, all was well, until a French 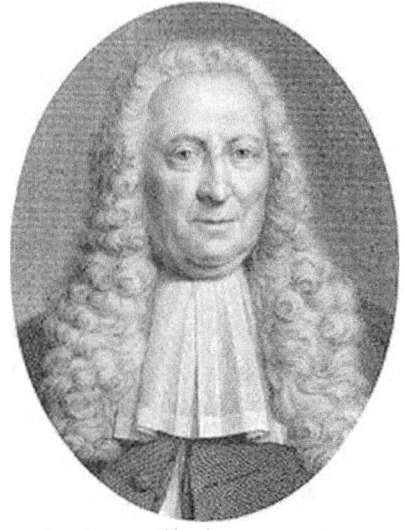 Naval Officer, named Gabriel Mathieu de Clieu, who was on leave from his station in Martinique, strolled into the court of King Louis XIV's and requested from the protective King, clippings from his beloved tree. Gabriel was summarily denied. Not to be dissuaded from his quest and certain that the Caribbean would be the perfect location for cultivating coffee, he would bide his time, playing out his role as charming guest of the court and enjoying all the merriment that was offered up, including liquor, numerous beautiful be-rouged and be-powdered women, who were clad in their finest, and at times, were seduced out of their finest by the handsome, irresistible Gabriel.

Patiently he played the cordial guest, waiting for his moment, for when the waning moon rose, Gabriel set out on the raid. He scaled the high walls of the Royal Botanical Garden, entered the hothouse, and then with history within his grasp he quickly snatched a cutting from the rare tree and made his way hastily to a waiting vessel! The ship was set to sail immediately, back to the French colony of Martinique in the West Indies.

On this fateful journey, Gabriel kept the little sprout below deck in a glass cabinet. Every day he tended to the precious treasure in his charge. He would bring it out to soak up the sun's rays, then back down to its protective quarters. Days passed into weeks, when suddenly a crew man on board with a devious plot (allegedly one with a Dutch accent), pulled a dagger out and fought vigorously with Gabriel to steal the cutting away. The Dutchman managed to break off a side-shoot, however Gabriel, with sword in hand prevailed, making the loathsome crewman submit to his will. The would-be thief was placed in shackles and later he most likely became fish food.

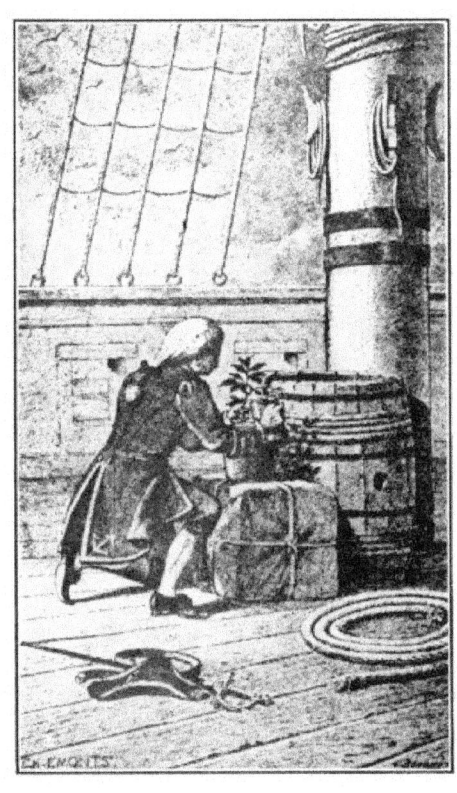

Days would pass and just when the journey seemed on fair sail, a savage attack by pirates took the crew a full day to fend off. By fates' will, they saved themselves and the priceless cargo below. And if all that wasn't enough for Gabriel and the coffee sprout, a horrendous storm nearly sent the ship to the bottom! The glass cabinet that housed the precious cargo was shattered and the limited fresh water supply nearly all lost. For the remainder of the journey, Gabriel shared his ration of water with his now wilting plant. Soon Martinique appears on the horizon and port just ahead, awaiting their arrival.

Gabriel secretly cultivated the coffee plant, hiding it behind other native plants to shield it from unwelcome eyes. De Clieu planted the it in the rich, fertile soil of Martinique and had his men guard the precious plant which thrived and multiplied. Some twenty months passed until the first small harvest was ready. He distributed it among the island's doctors and other intellectuals. Within three years, coffee plantations spread all over Martinique and its sister islands of St. Dominique and Guadeloupe. Coffee harvests were so large in the Caribbean that King Louis XIV finally forgave Gabriel for his thievery and made him Governor of the Antilles. So, I suppose, in some circumstances crime actually does pay!

The little sprout that could... would become the progenitor of 19 million trees in Martinique over the next 50 years and was the stock from which coffee trees throughout the Carribean, South and Central America all originated. I ask you, could this not be considered the greatest heist ever?

In the year 1723 the intrigue continued, the Brazilian government decided coffee was in their future. As a guise, to settle a border dispute between French Guiana and Dutch Guiana, on South America's jungle-ridden northern coast, Brazil sent the handsome Colonel Francisco de Melo Palheta to arbitrate a compromise. Yet his real objective was to acquire the oh-so desirable coffee plant. After all his proactive and successful efforts to mend the peace, the French Governor refused to grant Palheta's simple request for coffee seedlings. The Governor's denial did not detour Francisco who had arrived with a very seductive back-up plan. You could say he was the 007 of his day. It was no secret the Governor vigorously guarded the plantations to prevent cultivation from spreading, however his

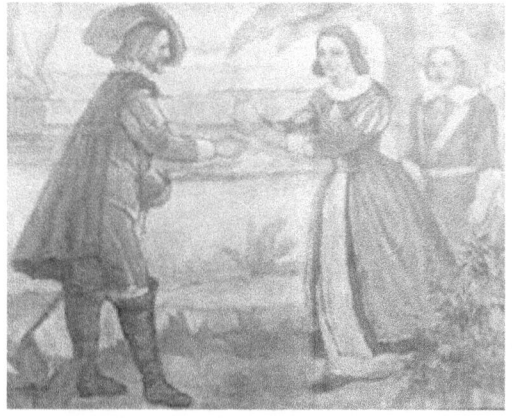

stunning wife, he did not guard so vigorously!

During a state dinner, the charming Francisco captivated the consideration of the beautiful Governor's wife. As they danced the night away, he whispered into her ear, "amore, amore, amore" tempting her with his Brazilian ways. The preoccupied Governor did not sense that his wife was about to give the farm away. After a secret liaison, the clandestine deal was sealed. As a bon voyage gift of appreciation and gratification, the French Governor's wife presents Francisco with a bouquet of flowers secretly sprinkled with her fertile coffee seedlings. From these cuttings grew the world's largest coffee empire we know today.

In the 1730's several momentous moments in coffee history took place. First in 1730, the former English Governor of Jamaica, Sir Nicolas Lawes, who is famous for prosecuting pirates, transported the first coffee plant to Jamaica. Cultivation soon started at the foothills of St. Andrew and quickly moved its way deep into the fertile Blue Mountains. While most of the coffee produced in Jamaica through the 18th century was traded throughout the world, it wasn't until coffee plantations were established in the Blue Mountain range that things took a turn for the extraordinary and Jamaica Blue Mountain coffee was first cultivated. Then, in 1732, In Germany, Johann Sebastian Bach got caught up in the coffee culture movement. He composed the hilarious "Coffee Cantata," and the lyrics. It's the story of a befuddled father who tries to get his headstrong, rebellious teenage daughter to kick the coffee habit and get married. It's a tough choice for her; coffee or marriage? Hmm...

The composition may very well have been inspired by a conversation Bach had with one of his own daughters. It was first performed in Zimmerman's Coffee House in Germany, where he often practiced and performed. Just read a few of the humorous lyrics that Bach wrote below:

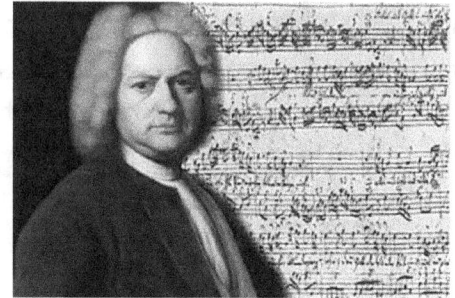

- **<u>Recitative Narrator</u>** - Be quiet, stop chattering, and pay attention to what's taking place: here comes Herr Schlendrian with his daughter Lieschen - he's growling like a honey bear. Hear for yourselves, what she has done to him!
- **<u>Aria – Schlendrian-</u>** Don't one's children cause one endless trials & tribulations! What I say each day to my daughter Lieschen falls on stony ground.
- **<u>Recitative – Schlendrian-</u>** You wicked child, you disobedient girl! When will I get my way; give up coffee!
- **<u>Lieschen-</u>** Father, don't be so severe! If I can't drink my bowl of coffee three times daily, then in my torment I will shrivel up like a piece of roast goat.
- **<u>Aria – Lieschen-</u>** Mmm! How sweet the coffee tastes, more delicious than a thousand kisses, mellower than muscatel wine. Coffee, coffee I must have, and if someone wishes to give me a treat, ah, then pour me out some coffee!
- **<u>Recitative – Schlendrian-</u>** If you don't give up drinking coffee then you shan't go to any wedding feast, nor go out walking. Oh! When will I get my way; give up coffee!
- **<u>Lieschen-</u>** Oh well! Just leave me my coffee!
- **<u>Schlendrian-</u>** Now I've got the little minx! I won't get you a whalebone skirt in the latest fashion.
- **<u>Lieschen-</u>** I can easily live with that.
- **<u>Schlendrian-</u>** You're not to stand at the window and watch people pass by!

- **Lieschen-** That as well, only I beg of you, leave me my coffee!
- **Schlendrian-** Furthermore, you shan't be getting any silver or gold ribbon for your bonnet from me!
- **Lieschen-** Yes, yes! Only leave me to my pleasure!
- **Schlendrian-** You disobedient Lieschen you, so you go along with it all!
- **Aria – Schlendrian-** Hard-hearted girls are not so easily won over. Yet if one finds their weak spot, ah! Then one comes away successful.
- **Recitative – Schlendrian-** Now take heed what your father says!
- **Lieschen-** In everything but the coffee.
- **Schlendrian-** Well then, you'll have to resign yourself to never taking a husband.
- **Lieschen-** Oh yes! Father, a husband!
- **Schlendrian-** I swear it won't happen.
- **Lieschen-** Until I can forgo coffee? From now on, coffee, remain forever untouched! Father, listen, I won't drink any.
- **Schlendrian-** Then you shall have a husband at last!
- **Aria – Lieschen-** Today even dear father, see to it! Oh, a husband! Really, that suits me splendidly! If it could only happen soon that at last, before I go to bed, instead of coffee I were to get a proper lover!
Recitative – Narrator- Old Schlendrian goes off to see if he can find a husband forthwith for his daughter Lieschen; but Leischen secretly lets it be known: no suitor is to come to my house unless he promises me, and it is also written into the marriage contract, that I will be permitted to make myself coffee whenever I want.

- **Trio-** A cat won't stop from catching mice, and maidens remain faithful to their coffee. The mother holds her coffee dear, the grandmother drank it also, who can thus rebuke the daughters!

Hilarious! But okay, back to coffee…

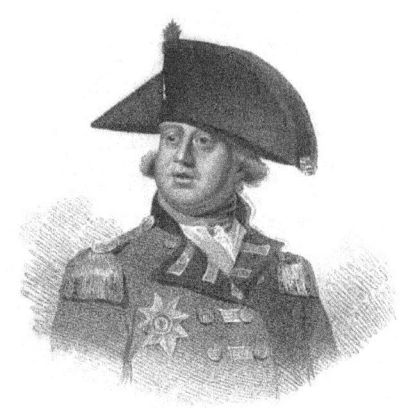

1773 and back in the New World, England's King George III imposed a heavy tax on tea, angering the people of Boston, who, as a protest against the unrepresented taxation of tea in America, rose up and took a first step towards independence, rejecting King George and the English. Meeting in the Green Dragon coffee house (which is still open today), the plan was set. The rebellious colonists dressed up as Native American Indians, snuck on-board ships in the harbor and threw the tea overboard. The Boston Tea Party made drinking coffee a patriotic duty. The Boston citizens who participate in this "Boston Tea Party" were still very angry over the 1765 Stamp Act crisis, and their renewed protests were the beginning of a major shift from tea to coffee as the predominant beverage of choice among the American people. Indeed, drinking coffee became an open expression of freedom. Before this time the wealthier classes were the main coffee drinkers while the less prosperous consumed tea, but with the events of 1773 that completely changed.

Next onto the revolution! Coffee kind of took a back seat to the War during this time as the whole world held its breath waiting to learn the outcome of the American Revolution.

In 1777, Frederick the Great of Prussia banned green coffee imports due to the decline of Prussia's wealth.

"It is disgusting to notice the increase in the quantity of coffee used by my subjects, and the amount of money that goes out of the country as a consequence. Everybody is using coffee; this must be prevented. His Majesty was brought up on beer, and so were both his ancestors and officers. Many battles have been fought and won by soldiers nourished on beer, and the King does not believe that coffee-drinking soldiers can be relied upon to endure hardships in case of another war." Due again to public outcry, thankfully, he was quickly forced to abandon the policy. The people would have their coffee!

1790 and back in the newly born United States of America, something else was brewing! In New York City, where the "Birthplace of our Union," was planned just 26 years earlier by Revolutionaries in the Merchants Coffee House, another revolution was first planned, this one economic: Well-heeled men sipped coffee while, for the first time, bought and sold public stock. In only two years, just across the street, the birth of the New York Stock Exchange took place. It was a beautiful spring day when a group of 24 men met outside of the Merchants Coffee House on Wall Street, in the shade of a huge sycamore tree that the locals called a "Buttonwood."

These far-sighted men, sipped their coffee while putting pen to parchment, and set down the rules which would govern the way they all agreed to conduct their trade; they called these rules the Buttonwood Agreement.

Later that same year, trading moved into a room on the second floor of the Tontine Coffee House where it remained until 1817. That building was eventually torn down, however its name carries on today on the New York high-rise in its place.

So, mankind moved into the nineteenth century as coffee's popularity and impact continued to grow. In 1817 Coffee cultivation was first introduced into Hawaii from Rio de Janeiro. Don Francisco de Paula Marin with the approval of King Kamehameha planted the first coffee seeds in Hawaii. The plantings were a failure but in 1825, the first successful coffee orchard was established. Kona coffee was soon to come!

Also in the early 1800s a Parisian named Laurens, a metal-smith, invented the first coffee percolator. And in 1822 just as George Stephenson was building the first steam-powered locomotive named 'locomotion', that would change the way we travel, kick off the industrial age and change the world forever, something even better and more important was starting to hiss.

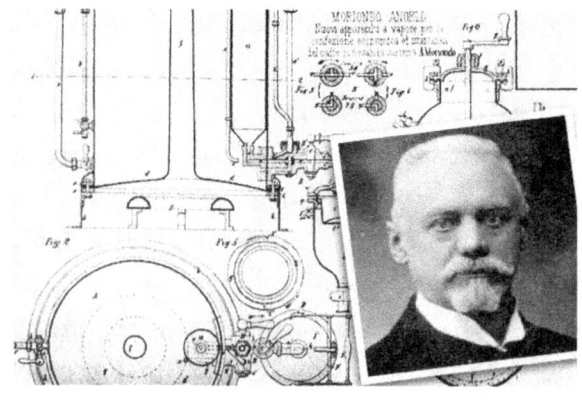

The world's first espresso machine steamed ahead in France. Louis Bernard Rabaut is credited with developing the brewing machine that used steam to force hot water through the coffee grounds, creating the first early version of what we know today as an Espresso machine! In the mid 1800 an American named James Mason, perfected the coffee percolator design.

Chapter 4: Coffee in America

Coffee, tea, and chocolate were introduced into North America almost simultaneously in the latter part of the seventeenth century. In the first half of the eighteenth century, tea had made such progress in England, thanks to the propaganda of the British East India Company, that, wanting to extend its use into the colonies, the directors turned their eyes in the direction of North America. Here, however, King George spoiled their well-laid plans by his unfortunate stamp act of 1765, which caused the colonists to raise the cry of "no taxation without representation."

Although the act was repealed in 1766, the right to tax was asserted, and in 1767 was again used, duties being laid on paints, oils, lead, glass, and tea. Once more the colonists resisted; and, by refusing to import any goods of English make, so distressed the English manufacturers that Parliament repealed every tax save that on tea. Despite the growing fondness for the beverage in America, the colonists preferred to get their tea elsewhere to sacrificing their principles and buying it from England. A brisk trade in smuggling tea from Holland was started.

In a panic at the loss of the most promising of its colonial markets, the British East India Company appealed to Parliament for aid, and was permitted to export tea, a privilege it had never before enjoyed. Cargoes were sent on consignment to selected commissioners in Boston, New York, Philadelphia, and Charleston. The story of the subsequent happenings properly belongs in a book on tea. It is sufficient here to refer to the climax of the agitation against the fateful tea tax, because it is undoubtedly responsible for our becoming a nation of coffee drinkers instead of one of tea drinkers, like England.

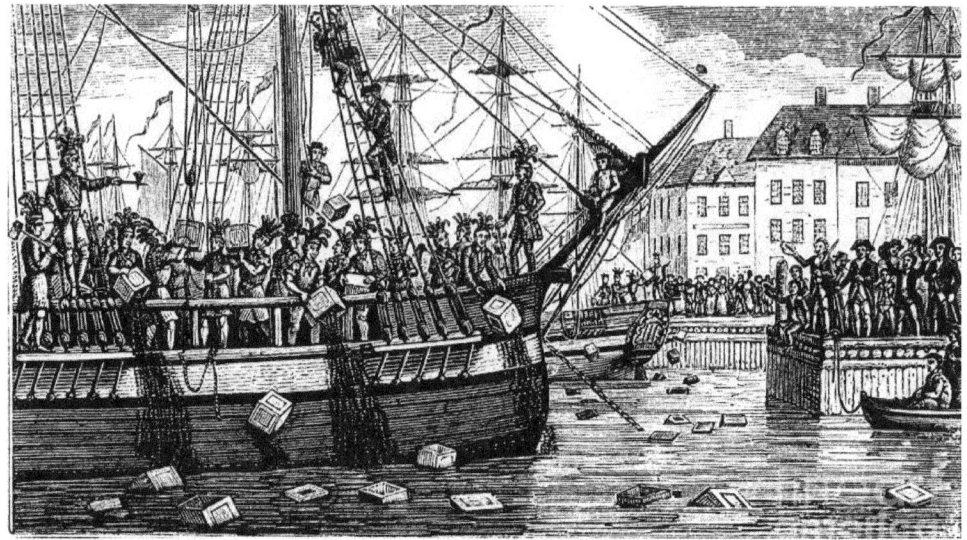

The Boston "tea party" of 1773, when citizens of Boston, disguised as Indians, boarded the English ships lying in Boston harbor and threw their tea cargoes into the bay, cast the die for coffee; for there and then originated a subtle prejudice against "the cup that cheers." Meanwhile, the change wrought in our social customs by this act, and those of like nature following it, in the New York, Pennsylvania, and Charleston colonies, caused coffee to be crowned "king of the American breakfast table", and the sovereign drink of the American people.

The history of coffee in colonial New England is so closely interwoven with the story of the inns and taverns that it is difficult to distinguish the genuine coffee house, as it was known in England, from the public house where lodgings and liquors were to be had. The coffee drink had strong competition from the heady wines, the liquors, and imported teas, and consequently it did not attain the vogue among the colonial New Englanders that it did among Londoners of the late seventeenth and early eighteenth centuries.

Although New England had its coffee houses, these were actually taverns where coffee was only one of the beverages served to patrons. They were generally meeting places for those who were conservative in their views regarding church and state, being friends of the ruling administration.

Most of the coffee houses were established in Boston, the metropolis of the Massachusetts Colony, and the social center of New England. While Plymouth, Salem, Chelsea, and Providence had taverns that served coffee, they did not achieve the name and fame of some of the more celebrated coffee houses in Boston. It is not definitely known when the first coffee was brought in; but it is reasonable to suppose that it came as part of the household supplies of some settler (probably between 1660 and 1670), who had become acquainted with it before leaving England. Or it may have been introduced by some British officer, who in London had made the rounds of the more celebrated coffee houses of the latter half of the seventeenth century.

According to early town records of Boston, Dorothy Jones was the first to be licensed to sell "coffee and cuchaletto," the latter being the seventeenth-century spelling for chocolate or cocoa. This license is dated 1670, and is said to be the first written reference to coffee in the Massachusetts Colony. It is not stated whether Dorothy Jones was a vender of the coffee drink or of "coffee powder," as ground coffee was known in the early days. There is some question as to whether Dorothy Jones was the first to sell coffee as a beverage in Boston. Londoners had known and drunk coffee for eighteen years before Dorothy Jones got her coffee license. British government officials were frequently taking ship from London to the

Massachusetts Colony, and it is likely that they brought tidings and samples of the coffee the English gentry had lately taken up. No doubt they also told about the new-style coffee houses that were becoming popular in all parts of London. And it may be assumed that their tales caused the landlords of the inns and taverns of colonial Boston to add coffee to their lists of beverages.

Of course, coffee was not only taking hold in Boston. The Dutch, the founders of New York, seem to have introduced tea into New Amsterdam before they brought in coffee. This was somewhere about the middle of the seventeenth century. We find it recorded that about 1668 the burghers succumbed to coffee. Coffee made its way slowly, first in the homes, where it replaced the "must", or beer, at breakfast. Chocolate came about the same time, but was more of a luxury than tea or coffee.

After the surrender of New York to the British in 1674, English manners and customs were rapidly introduced. First tea, and later coffee, were favorite beverages in the homes. By 1683 New York had become so central a market for the green bean, that William Penn, as soon as he found himself comfortably settled in the Pennsylvania Colony, sent over to New York for his coffee supplies. It was not long before a social need arose that only the London style of coffee house could fill.

The coffee houses of early New York, like their prototypes in London, Paris, and other old world capitals, were the centers of the business, political and, to some extent, of the social life of the city. But they never became the forcing-beds of literature that the French and English houses were, principally because the colonists had no professional writers of any real note.

There is one outstanding feature of the early American coffee houses, particularly of those opened in New York, that is not distinctive of the European houses. The colonists sometimes held court trials in the long, or assembly, room of the early coffee houses; and often held their general assembly and council meetings there.

The early coffee house was an important factor in New York life. What the perpetuation of this public gathering place meant to the citizens is shown by a complaint (evidently designed to revive the declining fortunes of the historic Merchants coffee house) in the *New York Journal* of October 19, 1775, which, in part, said:

To the Inhabitants of New York:
It gives me concern, in this time of public difficulty and danger, to find we have in this city no place of daily general meeting, where we might hear and communicate intelligence from every quarter and freely confer with one another on every matter that concerns us. Such a place of general meeting is of very great advantage in many respects, especially at such a time as this, besides the satisfaction it affords and the sociable disposition it has a tendency to keep up among us, which was never more wanted than at this time. To answer all these and many other good and useful purposes, coffee houses have been universally deemed the most convenient places of resort, because, at a small expense of time or money, persons wanted may be found and spoke with, appointments may be made, current news heard, and whatever it most concerns us to know. In all cities, therefore, and large towns that I have seen in the British dominions, sufficient encouragement has been given to support one or more coffee houses in a genteel manner. How comes it then that New York, the most central, and one of the largest and most prosperous cities in British America, cannot support one coffee house? It is a scandal to the city and its inhabitants to be destitute of such a convenience for want of due encouragement. A coffee house, indeed, there is, a very good and comfortable one, extremely well-tended and

accommodated, but it is frequented but by an inconsiderable number of people; and I have observed with surprise, that but a small part of those who do frequent it, contribute anything at all to the expense of it, but come in and go out without calling for or paying anything to the house. In all the coffee houses in London, it is customary for every one that comes in to call for at least a dish of coffee, or leave the value of one, which is but reasonable, because when the keepers of these houses have been at the expense of setting them up and providing all necessaries for the accommodation of company, every one that comes to receive the benefit of these conveniences ought to contribute something towards the expense of them.

Some chroniclers of New York's early days are confident that the first coffee house in America was opened in New York; but the earliest authenticated record they have presented is that on November 1, 1696, John Hutchins bought a lot on Broadway, between Trinity churchyard and what is now Cedar Street, and there built a house, naming it the King's Arms. Against this record, the citizens of Boston can present, in Samuel Gardner Drake's *History and Antiquities of the City of Boston* that Benjamin Harris sold books at the "London Coffee House" in 1689. I really do not think that it matters who was first, I think that what matters is that we understand that coffee has been a part of American culture and custom since before the founding of the United States.

The city of Philadelphia was not left out of the coffee house craze. William Penn is generally credited with the introduction of coffee into the Quaker colony which he founded on the Delaware in 1682. He also brought to the "city of brotherly love" that other great drink of human brotherhood, tea. At first, in the early 1700s, like tea, coffee was only a drink for the well-to-do. As was the case in the other English colonies, coffee languished for a time while tea rose in favor, more especially in the home.

Following the stamp act of 1765, and the tea tax of 1767, the Pennsylvania Colony joined hands with the others in a general tea boycott; and coffee received the same impetus as elsewhere in the colonies that became the thirteen original states.

The coffee houses of early Philadelphia loom large in the history of the city and the republic. Picturesque in themselves, with their distinctive colonial architecture, their associations also were romantic. Many a civic, sociological, and industrial reform came into existence in the low-ceilinged, sanded-floor main rooms of the city's early coffee houses.

For many years, 'Ye coffee house', the two 'London coffee houses', and the' City tavern' (also known as the 'Merchants coffee house') each in its turn dominated the official and social life of Philadelphia. The earlier houses were the regular meeting places of Quaker municipal officers, ship captains, and merchants who came to transact public and private business. As the outbreak of the Revolution drew near, fiery colonials, many in Quaker garb, congregated there to argue against British oppression of the colonies. After the Revolution, the leading citizens resorted to the coffee house to dine and sup and to hold their social functions.

When the city was founded in 1682, coffee cost too much to admit of its being retailed to the general public at coffee houses. William Penn wrote in his *Accounts* that in 1683 coffee in the berry was sometimes procured in New York at a cost of eighteen shillings nine pence the pound, equal to about $4.68. He also mentions that meals were served in the ordinaries at six pence (equal to twelve cents), to wit: "We have seven ordinaries for the entertainment of strangers and for workmen that are not housekeepers, and a good meal is to be had there for six pence sterling." With green coffee costing $4.68 a pound, making the price of a cup about seventeen cents, it is not likely that coffee was on the menus of the ordinaries serving meals at twelve cents each. Ale was the common meal-time beverage.

There were four classes of public houses—inns, taverns, ordinaries, and coffee houses. The inn was a modest hotel that supplied lodgings, food, and drink, the beverages consisting mostly of ale, port, Jamaica rum, and Madeira wine. The tavern, though accommodating guests with bed and board, was more of a drinking place than a lodging house. The ordinary combined the characteristics of a restaurant and a boarding house. The coffee house was a pretentious tavern, dispensing, in most cases, intoxicating drinks as well as coffee.

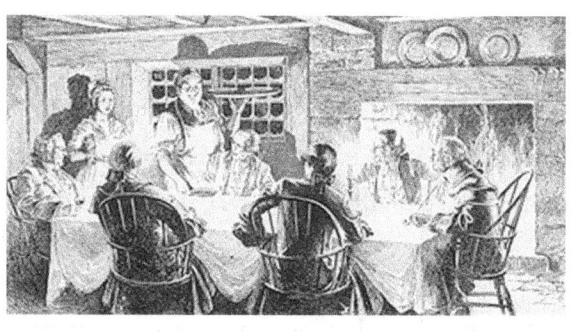

The first house of public resort opened in Philadelphia bore the name of the Blue Anchor tavern, and was probably established in 1683 or 1684; colonial records do not state definitely. As its name indicates, this was a tavern. The first coffee house came into existence about the year 1700. Watson, in one place in his *Annals* of the city, says 1700, but in another 1702. The earlier date is thought to be correct, and is seemingly substantiated by the co-authors Scharf and Westcott in their *History* of the city, in which they say, "The first public house designated as a coffee house was built in Penn's time [1682–1701] by Samuel Carpenter, on the east side of Front Street, probably above Walnut Street. That it was the first of its kind—the only one in fact for some years—seems to be established beyond doubt. It was always referred to in old times as 'Ye Coffee House.'"

Chapter 5: Coffee Goes to War

It is not stretching the truth to say that coffee played an important role in the founding of this country. From its introduction to European culture, coffee had been considered synonymous with intellectual discourse. Because of the connection between coffee and politics, it is perhaps the most important drink for American history.

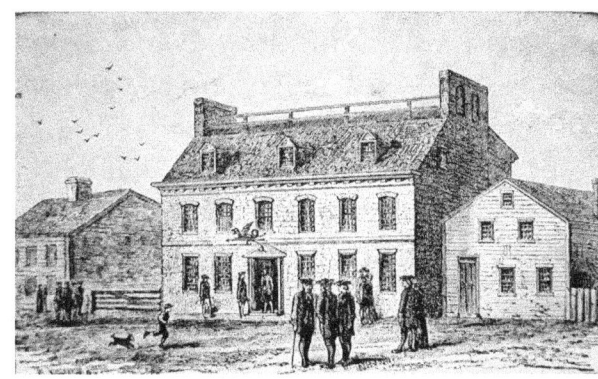

The great thinkers of the 18th Century would gather at colonial coffee houses/taverns, such as the Green Dragon in Boston, to discuss the important issues of the time. In 1765, a crowd gathered to burn an effigy of Andrew Oliver. Oliver was doing the unpopular work of King George III by selling stamps, a form of taxation. The group eventually dispersed, but they gathered the next day at the Green Dragon to discuss the political events of the previous day. In so doing, they formed a group that they dubbed the Sons of Liberty. The Green Dragon Inn, Tavern and Coffee House was their regular meeting place.

When the British sought to punish the colonies by unfair taxation on tea, coffee became not only the preferred drink, but the patriotic one as well. The East India Company couldn't conceive of the colonists doing without tea, so they sent over a full cargo of tea in a marketing scheme that would pay the taxes to the King, but cut out the middlemen merchants. This scheme infuriated the colonists. A particularly energized group in Boston carried out the event which became known as the Boston Tea Party. They threw tea overboard and vowed against drinking tea, in favor of coffee.

With the advent of the Revolutionary War, coffee houses soon became the preferred meeting place of the newly formed Continental Congress. The most famous coffee house of the time was the Merchant's Coffee House in Philadelphia. It was there where the Declaration of Independence was first read aloud to the public.

One could argue that America began to define itself by its connection with coffee as opposed to tea. So, stand up for something you believe in, drink coffee and make our forefathers proud! On July 4th, 1776, the Continental Congress ratified the Declaration of Independence. This incredible document written by our founding fathers gave America its direction and has shaped our politics ever since. Every July 4th, we celebrate our independence from the colonial rule of Great Britain. We celebrate American freedom. However, what many people may not know is how influential coffee was in the revolution.

As mentioned earlier, coffee, the lesser-consumed beverage at the time prior to the Boston Tea Party, became the patriotic drink of choice for revolutionaries after the event. Loyalists still continued to enjoy their tea and unbeknownst to them, this put them, and the British, at an intelligence disadvantage.

You see, the movers and shakers of the Revolution began meeting in coffee houses to talk about politics and freedom. The coffee houses were not friendly places for the loyalists to find themselves, so they stayed far away. Avoiding the coffee houses meant that they did not know exactly what the rabble rousers were getting up to, they had no inkling of the plans that were being hatched.

The unique culture that sprang up in the coffee houses allowed people to meet without the threat of the tea-loving British overhearing the revolutionaries' plans. This provided the time and space for the Declaration of Independence to be crafted without fear of punishment. Thus, coffee became a symbol of hope and freedom. Coffee's tradition of freedom and hope continues today with the rise of the Fairtrade, Direct-Trade, and other ethical sourcing practices. Coffee, when sourced with equity, continues to change the world from tyranny to liberty.

Coffee was eagerly embraced by the patriots of the day as it showed a symbolic rejection of the English practice of drinking tea. This sentiment became so pervasive that Coffee was declared the National Drink of the Colonized United States by the Continental Congress.

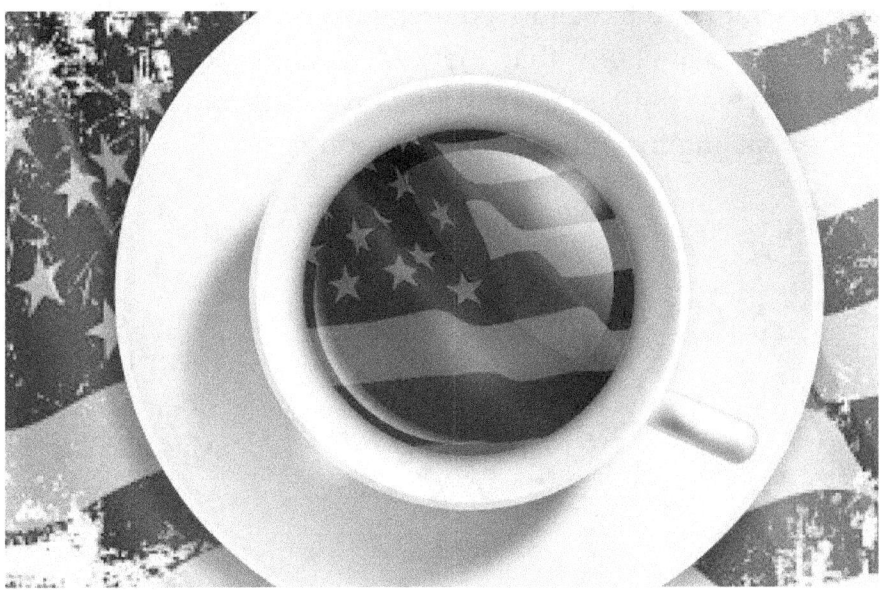

Coffee remained popular, but it was the embargo of the tea trade by Britain following the War of 1812 that cemented America's relationship with daily coffee. During this time coffee became a part of American Culture that has endured to today.

In 1860, after deciding against heading to the gold-filled streams in the Sierra mountains and participating in California's 1849 gold rush, James Folger worked in San Francisco, where its Barbary Coast was filled with saloons and scantily-clad women in bordellos, who kept men up all night long. He soon hit gold of his own when he founded the J.A. Folger Coffee Company. He was a pioneer in west coast coffee and helped create the California caffeine rush that worked to keep those 49er prospectors digging, and those other hung-over newcomers building the great state that California was soon to become.

Also in the 1860s, Jabez Burns of New York, was granted a United States patent on the original Burns coffee roaster, the first machine which did not have to be moved away from the fire for discharging roasted coffee, and one that marked a major advance for coffee roasting. He was the Thomas Edison of roasting and the grandfather of all the roasting machines we know today!

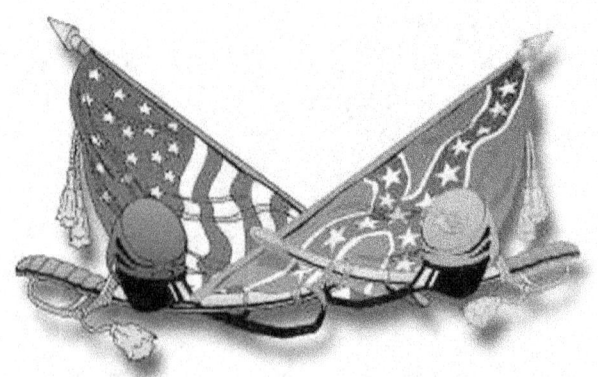

The 1860s also saw the American Civil War break out. Coffee was a favorite on both sides of the Mason-Dixon line. Loved by both the Blue and the Gray!

One incredible story from those war years concerns a young man named Billy, and it was to become known as one of the greatest coffee runs in American history! You see, few things are as welcome to soldiers in camp or on the march, as a cup of fresh, hot, coffee. Somewhere amid the horror and bloodshed of one battle, a small act of kindness was rendered that would be remembered decades later.

The battle had begun before daylight, leaving harried soldiers no time for breakfast. By that afternoon, the Ohio boys had been fighting since morning, trapped in the raging battle of Antietam, in September of 1862. Late in the afternoon a 19-year-old commissary sergeant with Company E, 23rd Ohio Infantry, decided he had to do something to ease the suffering of his comrades on the front lines. Bravely exposing himself to barrage after barrage of Confederate fire, he organized a mobile field kitchen and dodged bullets to move it up and down the line so that he could serve warm food and hot coffee to the suffering troops.

Today a monument at Antietam commemorates Billy's battlefield service and includes a panel depicting him handing a cup of coffee to an exhauster soldier. As much as it is a memorial to that brave young soldier, it can also be seen as a monument to coffee, which was held in tremendous esteem during the war. As Billy scurried from position to position the men held out tin cups, gulped the brew and started fighting again. "It was like putting a new regiment in the fight," their officer recalled. It made a real difference. Three decades later, Billy, that much appreciated coffee boy, rode that singular act of caffeinated heroism straight into the White House, for you see, it turned out that Billy, the brave 19-year-old coffee boy the grateful troops never forgot, was none other than William McKinley, who became the 25th President of the United States.

At the time, no one found William McKinley's act all that strange. For Union soldiers, and the lucky Confederates who could scrounge some, coffee fueled the war. Soldiers drank it before marches, after marches, on patrol, during combat. In their diaries, "coffee" appears more frequently than the words "rifle," "cannon" or "bullet." Ragged veterans and tired nurses agreed with one diarist: "Nobody can 'soldier' without coffee."

Union troops made their coffee everywhere, and with everything: with water from canteens and puddles, brackish bays and Mississippi mud, liquid their horses would not drink. They cooked it over the fires of plundered fence rails, or heated mugs in scalding steam-vents on naval gunboats. When times were good, coffee accompanied beefsteaks and oysters; when they were bad it washed down raw salt-pork and maggoty hardtack. Coffee was often the last comfort troops enjoyed before entering battle, and the first sign of safety for those who survived. The Union Army encouraged this love, issuing soldiers roughly 36 pounds of coffee each year. Men ground the beans themselves and brewed it in little pots called 'muckets.' They spent much of their downtime discussing the quality of that morning's brew. Reading their diaries, one can sense the delight (and addiction) as troops gushed about a "delicious cup of black," or fumed about "wishy-washy coffee." Escaped slaves who joined Union Army camps could always find work as cooks if they were good at "settling" the coffee – getting the grounds to sink to the bottom of the unfiltered muckets.

For much of the war, the massive Union Army of the Potomac made up the second-largest population center in the Confederacy, and each morning this sprawling city became a coffee factory. First, as another diarist noted, "little campfires, rapidly increasing to hundreds in number, would shoot up along the hills and plains."

Then the encampment buzzed with the sound of thousands of grinders simultaneously crushing beans. Soon tens of thousands of muckets gurgled with fresh brew.

Confederates were not so lucky. The Union blockade kept most coffee out of seceded territory. One British observer noted that the loss of coffee "afflicts the Confederates even more than the loss of spirits," while an Alabama nurse joked that the fierce craving for caffeine would, somehow, be the Union's "means of subjugating us." When coffee was available, captured or smuggled or traded with Union troops during casual cease-fires, Confederates wrote rhapsodically about their first sip. But the Rebel's problem spilled over to the Union invaders, too. When Gen. William T. Sherman's Union troops decided to live off plunder and forage as they cut their way through Georgia and South Carolina, soldiers complained that while food was plentiful, there were no beans to be found. "Coffee is only got from Uncle Sam," an Ohio officer grumbled, and his men "could scarce get along without it."

Yes, Civil War soldiers on both sides loved their coffee. It was, after all, one of the few items in a soldier's food ration that was both reliable and highly coveted. Between half-rotten meat and iron-tough bread, the Union food ration was often a disappointment, "Sore feet an' damned short rations, that's all," a soldier laments in Stephen Crane's *The Red Badge of Courage*—a common complaint. Coffee, by contrast, tended to hold up well in a soldier's pack and was appreciated whenever it could be consumed.

"Coffee was one of the most cherished items in the ration," wrote Bell Irvin Wiley in his classic *The Life of Billy Yank*, published in 1952. "The effect on morale must have been considerable. And if it cannot be said that coffee helped Billy Yank win the war, it at least made his participation in the conflict more tolerable."

Coffee's power had been known around the world for centuries. It was prepared and drunk with reverence in the Middle East and Africa from the 15th century on. By the 17th century, the caffeinated beverage had spread throughout the western world. After the Boston Tea Party, John Adams declared that "tea must be universally renounced." In its wake, coffee flourished.

So addictive was this elixir that the Sioux called it *kazuta sapa*— "black medicine." The early 19th century also brought technological innovations such as a two-tier drip pot invented in France, according to Mark Pendergrast, author of *Uncommon Grounds: The History of Coffee and How it Transformed the World*. In 1850 young entrepreneur Jim Folger opened a coffee-roasting business in San Francisco, planting the seeds of a coffee empire. Coffee had become, according to Lieutenant William H.C. Whiting, a 19th-century Army engineer, "the great essential in a prairie bill of fare."

Before the war, New Orleans was the primary port for the coffee trade in the United States, with the most popular suppliers coming from Java, Ceylon, Brazil and Costa Rica—the great irony being that the coffee industry in many places, such as Brazil, relied on slave labor or horrific working conditions. The Southern port was quickly superseded by New York after the blockade was put in place. Coffee prices steadily increased as the war went on; the price of Brazilian coffee jumped from 14 cents a pound in 1861 to a high of 42 cents a pound by war's end. That was nothing compared to the $5 per pound price found in the South, which sometimes went much higher. In 1832 President Andrew Jackson added coffee to the official military food ration, where it remains today (although the coffee is instant in today's MREs). At the outbreak of the Civil War, the Union food ration included 12 ounces of pork or bacon, one pound and 4 ounces of salt or fresh beef, flour or bread, corn, beans or peas, and coffee. Coffee beans were usually distributed whole and roasted, although green beans were often dispensed as well. (An attempt to distribute canned instant coffee known as "essence of coffee", a coffee extract mixed with milk and sugar, was short-lived.) By 1864, the U.S. government was purchasing 40 million pounds of coffee beans.

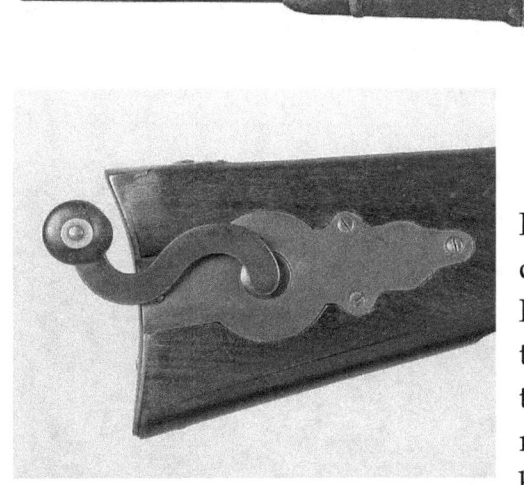

Preparation was time-consuming but straightforward. First soldiers roasted the beans if they were green, then ground the roasted beans with a rock or rifle butt when it came time to brew. By the end of the war, some Sharps Carbines had been modified to include a hand-cranked grinder for coffee or grain, though existing examples of these are extremely rare. The grounds and water were put together in a pot and brought to a boil over a fire. Before drinking, soldiers either strained the grounds through a piece of cloth or let the grounds settle to the bottom of their tin cups, skimming them off when needed. The drink was usually prepared black and "strong enough to float an iron wedge," according to F.Y. Hedley of the 32nd Illinois, and soldiers learned to drink it straight (without milk), although sugar was often added whenever it was available. One common technique among veterans was to mix the sugar evenly throughout their coffee beans before brewing, so as to never be caught without a sweetened cup. Some had been told to use such items as eggshells or fish to "clarify" the drink, but it's doubtful that the resulting taste or extra steps involved gained widespread use in the field.

It wasn't long before coffee began to show up in the literature and art of the period. In 1863 Winslow Homer published six lithographs in a volume called *Campaign Sketches*, which his publisher sold as a set of "spirited Camp scenes" for just $1.50. Homer's sketches ranged from the sentimental ("The Letter for Home") to the comical ("Foraging," starring a runaway cow), but one image above all captured the daily grind of war, literally: "The Coffee Call."

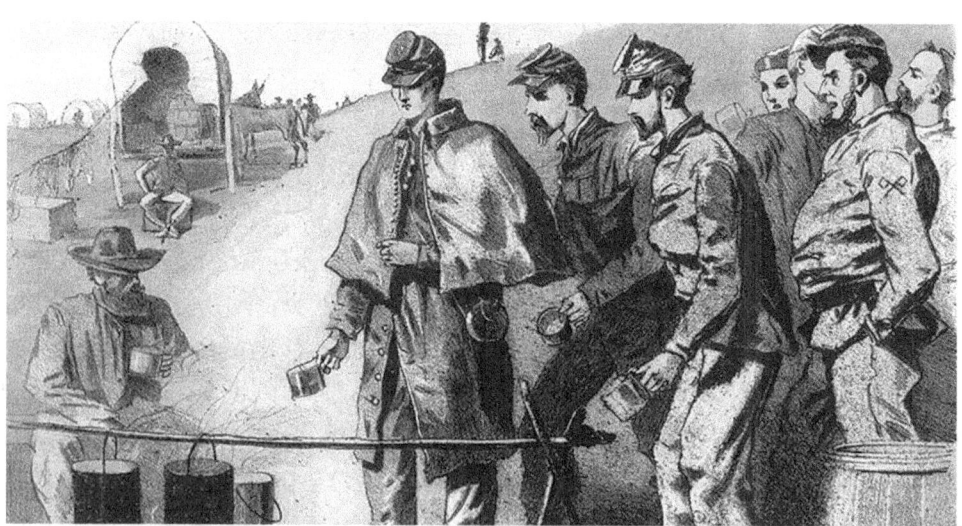

Chilly troops line up for a warm cup of Joe in Winslow Homer's print "The Coffee Call."
Library of Congress.

In Homer's sketch, above, several soldiers with tin cups in hand, and including one wearing a long greatcoat (indicating cold weather), eagerly await coffee brewing in two pots over an open flame. Sometime during the war, artist Alfred Waud, best known for his battle drawings for *Harper's Weekly*, drew a hasty sketch of a bearded soldier with a scribbled title, "The Veteran Coffee Boiler." He also added a first-person caption in the margin (original spelling and punctuation retained): *"Now they are going to have another fight I ain't spoiling for a fight But I don't see any help for it, I've boiled coffee till I have got no more, my rations are about played out and I never see sich a mean country a chip bird might starve if he did not move out quick. Weel I'll go and fire off these cartridges."*

The business of coffee was captured in photographs too. Timothy H. O'Sullivan, who had taken a famous photo of Waud at Devil's Den at Gettysburg during 1863, made a stereograph in 1864 of African-American soldiers brewing coffee in front of a bombproof at Petersburg, capturing troops enjoying a rare and refreshing break

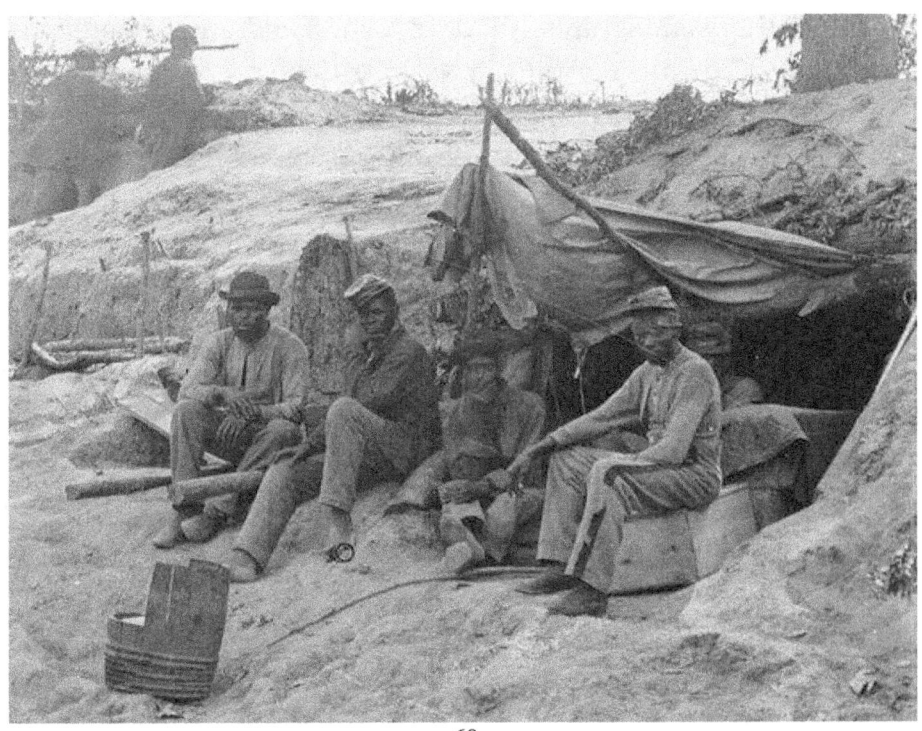

from some of the conflict's most brutal fighting. The photo is presented on the previous page.

"Whatever words of condemnation or criticism may have been bestowed on other government rations," wrote Union veteran John D. Billings in his classic 1888 work on the subject, *Hard Tack and Coffee*, "there was but one opinion of the coffee that was served out, and that was of unqualified acceptance." A veteran of the 10th Massachusetts Artillery, Billings acknowledged that coffee had been given second billing in his title, noting, "Some old veterans may be disposed to question the judgment which gives it this rank, and claim that coffee should take first place." He argued that, while bread or hardtack provided actual sustenance, coffee was merely a stimulant. Its stimulating effects were nonetheless treasured. "What a Godsend it seemed to us at times!" Billings wrote. "How often after being completely jaded by a night march, and this was an experience common to thousands, have I had a wash, if there was water to be had, made and drunk my pint or so of coffee and felt as fresh and invigorated as if just arisen from a night's sound sleep!"

As much as coffee was admired, its quality depended greatly on who was brewing it. One Irish soldier, according to Wiley, said the coffee prepared by company cooks in large pots was indistinguishable from the company soup. He despised it so much that he had no choice but to drink "Adam's Ale instead," referring to water, the only drink available to Adam in the Garden of Eden. Coffee showed up regularly in diaries and letters home too. On May 19th, 1862, as his unit marched through northern Virginia, Franklin Eldredge of the 7th Ohio Infantry wrote about his routine: "Fine morning, started at eight…shaved, washed, and changed; we eat our 'Little John' ration of coffee and hard bread, when we are ordered to be ready to march immediately." A week later, according to his diary, a rainy day made it impossible for Eldredge and his comrades to get a fire going, so they were forced to "steep" their coffee instead of boiling it, "which tasted bully."

In his Civil War chronicle, *Corporal Si Klegg and His Pard*, Wilbur H. Hinman, former lieutenant colonel of the 65th Ohio Infantry, wrote that "it is safe to say that if forced to strike one [item] from the bill of fare, not one in a hundred would have marked out coffee. If hardtack or bacon ran short, it could be eked out with odds and ends picked up by foraging, but there was nothing to take the place of coffee."

Even if there was no real substitute for coffee, Confederates made the attempt anyway. When the Union blockade was in effect, the coffee trade in the South virtually dried up, forcing Southern soldiers and civilians to drink coffee substitutes that were, at best, weak approximations. Ernestine Weiss Faudie, a German immigrant who resided in Texas and whose two brothers fought for the Confederacy, said in an oral history that her family made a coffee substitute out of sweet potatoes. "We cut them up and dried them and boiled them," she said, "and 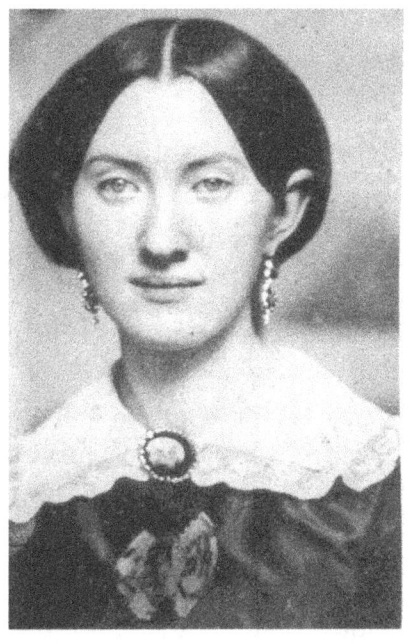 drank this for coffee." Others brewed tepid concoctions from peanuts, peas, dried fruit, acorns, corn, rye or chicory. One recipe called for cutting the roots of dandelions into small pieces, roasting them until crisp, and grinding them up. If they were lucky, Southerners could mix these impostors with real coffee grounds, stretching their supply.

In 1861 one R.J. Dawson wrote out a "receipt" (recipe) for beet coffee and sent it to the *Chronicle & Sentinel* of Augusta, Ga.:

"Take the common garden beet, wash it clean, cut it up into small pieces, twice the size of a grain of coffee; put into the coffee toaster or oven, and roast as you do your coffee—perfectly brown...

When sufficiently dry and hard, grind it in a clean mill, and take half a common sized coffee cup of the grounds, and boil with one gallon water. Then settle with an egg, and send to the table, hot. Sweeten with very little sugar, and add good cream or milk."

Dawson added that the coffee *"can be drank by children, with impunity, and will not (in my judgment) either impair sight or nerves."* He added, *"Try it, as an antidote to the blockade."*

Confederate soldiers and civilians would not go without. Many cooked up coffee substitutes, roasting corn or rye or chopped beets, grinding them finely and brewing up something warm and brown. It contained no caffeine, but desperate soldiers claimed to love it. Gen. George Pickett, famous for that failed charge at Gettysburg, thanked his wife for the delicious "coffee" she had sent, gushing: "No Mocha or Java ever tasted half so good as this rye-sweet-potato blend!" John Jacob Omenhausser, a Confederate soldier imprisoned at Camp Lookout, Md., between June 1864 and June 1865, produced a variety of often humorous watercolors of prison life. One of these, called *Coffee Grounds Collector*, depicts one Rebel soldier asking another, "Mr. has any one spoke for your coffee grounds?" When the other soldier graciously offers them up, the man says in relief: "Thank the lord I'm in luck once more." As much luck as an imprisoned soldier could have, at least.

Did the fact that Union troops were near jittery from coffee, while rebels survived on impotent brown water, have an impact on the outcome of the conflict? Union soldiers certainly thought so. Though they rarely used the word "caffeine," in their letters and diaries they raved about that "wonderful stimulant in a cup of coffee," considering it a "nerve tonic." One depressed soldier wrote home that he was surprised that he was still living, and reasoned: "what keeps me alive must be the coffee."

Others went further, considering coffee a weapon of war. Gen. Benjamin Butler ordered his men to carry coffee in their canteens, and planned attacks based on when his men would be most caffeinated. He assured another general, before a fight in October 1864, that "if your men get their coffee early in the morning you can hold."

Coffee alone, did not win the war – Union material resources and manpower played a much, much bigger role than the quality of its java – but it does say something about the victors. From one perspective, coffee was emblematic of the new Northern order of fast-paced wage labor, a hurried, business-minded, industrializing nation of strivers. For years, Northern bosses had urged their workers to switch from liquor to coffee, dreaming of sober, caffeinated, untiring employees. Southerners drank coffee too, in New Orleans especially, but the way Union soldiers gulped the stuff at every meal pointed the way toward the world that ugly war made, a civilization that lives on today in every office breakroom.

But more than that, coffee was simply delicious and soothing, "the soldier's chiefest bodily consolation" for men and women pushed beyond their limits. Caffeine was secondary. Soldiers often brewed coffee at the end of long marches, deep in the night while other men assembled tents. These soldiers were far too tired for caffeine to make much of a difference; they just wanted to share a warm cup, of

Brazilian beans or scorched rye, a moment of camaraderie, before passing out. This explains their fierce love of the "black gold". When one captured Union soldier was finally freed from a prison camp, he meditated on his experiences. Over his first cup of coffee in more than a year, he wondered if he could ever forgive "those Confederate thieves for robbing me of so many precious doses." Getting worked up, he fumed, "Just think of it, in three hundred days there was lost to me, forever, so many hundred pots of good old Government Java." So, when William McKinley, braved enemy fire to take his comrades each that warm "cup of Joe" he knew what it meant to every one of those future voters!

Whether it was drunk by the common soldier or a U.S. president, coffee was widely consumed through the end of the war. Years later, in 1887, Robert Todd Lincoln received a surprising gift from Captain D.W. Taylor in the form of a coffee cup. Taylor said that a White House servant had seen President Lincoln place the cup on a windowsill on the evening of April 14, 1865, before leaving for Ford's Theatre, and the servant saved it as a souvenir (the cup itself now belongs to the Smithsonian). There is some small comfort in knowing that coffee, so simple and yet so welcome, may have been the last thing the ill-fated president ever drank.

Following the Civil War in 1870, John Arbuckle, with the aid of a draftsman and machinist invented a machine that filled, weighed, sealed and labeled coffee in paper packages. From his factory in New York, the "Arbuckle Ariosa" became the first mass produced coffee sold all over the country. Eventually Arbuckle became the largest importer of coffee in the world and soon became the largest ship owner in America because every merchant ship engaged in the South American coffee trade was his.

In 1907 ★★ Theodore Roosevelt said
"Good to the Last Drop!"

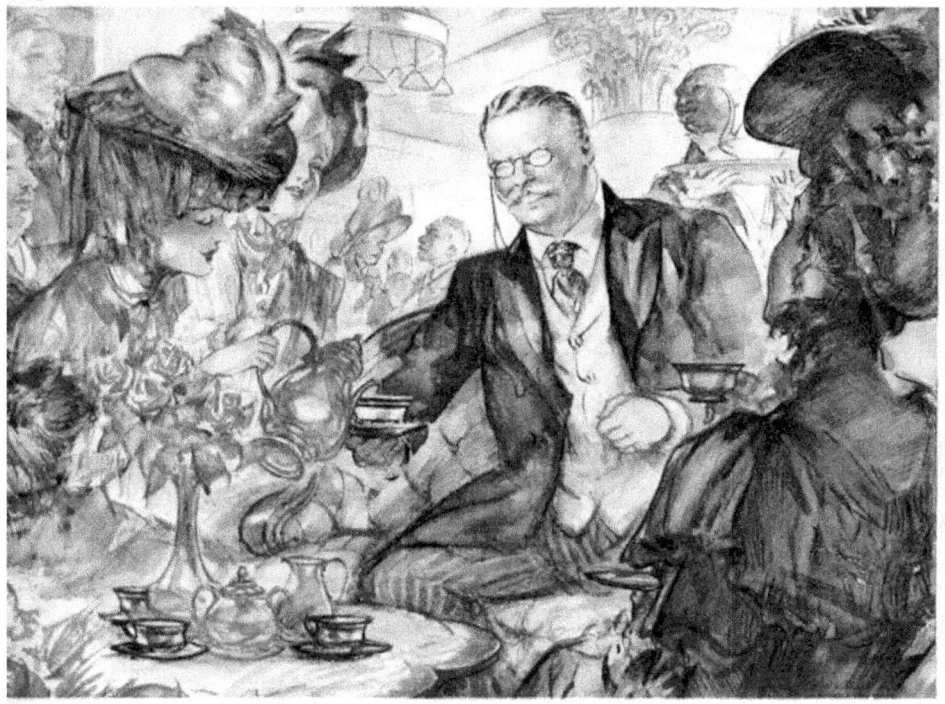

And now more than ever — These Words are True!
REAL COFFEE ENJOYMENT...YOU CAN COUNT ON MAXWELL HOUSE

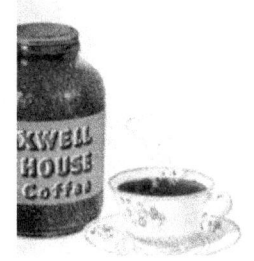

● To nearly every American, "Good to the Last Drop" means *good* coffee . . . *Maxwell House Coffee!* It's one of America's most famous slogans. *But* do you know how it began?

Back in 1907 President Theodore Roosevelt visited Nashville, Tennessee. There was an ovation for him—both in the famous old Maxwell House Hotel—and throughout the city. During this visit he enjoyed his first cup of Maxwell House Coffee, and when offered another cup the President exclaimed, "Delighted! It's *good to the last drop!*"

This gracious tribute caught the fancy of Mr. Joel Cheek, creator of the renowned Maxwell House blend. And so—a slogan was born!

As time went by, the fame of Maxwell House Coffee spread far and wide. Today it is enjoyed by *more people* than any other brand of coffee in the world for its friendly stimulation and extra flavor. Expertly blended for *richness, mellowness, full body,* and *vigor* . . . Radiant-Roasted to develop the full flavor goodness . . . it is now, more than ever, truly *"Good to the Last Drop!"*

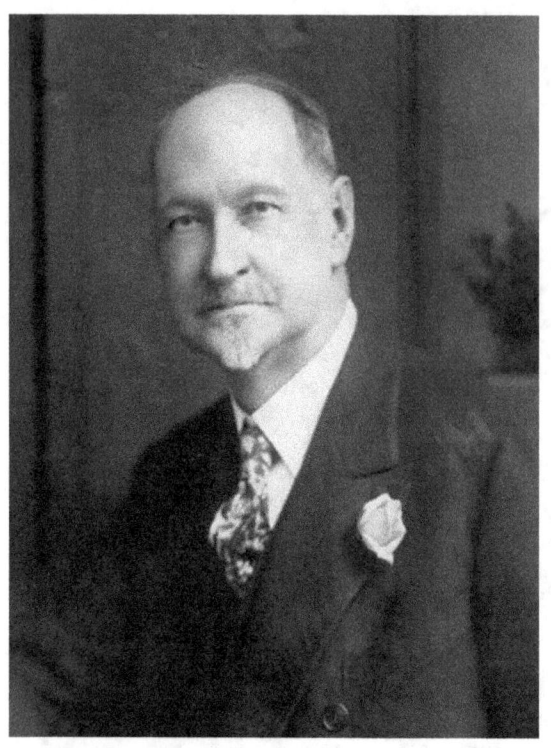

Then in 1886, a young fellow named Joel Cheek named his new coffee blend "Maxwell House" after the ritzy hotel that served it in Nashville, Tennessee. Seven presidents stayed at the Maxwell House Hotel, including Theodore Roosevelt, whose 1907 comment that this delightful coffee was "Good to the Last Drop" launched the advertising slogan that was used to promote the nation's first blended coffees. You can see one of those first ads on the next page.

Chapter 6: 20ᵗʰ Century Coffee

Well, the wars of early American history and the 1800s were over and mankind along with our favorite morning beverage moved into the Twentieth Century. And that turn of the century provided a Happy New Year for coffee, and for a couple of brothers. The Hills Brothers packaged roasted coffee beans for the first time using vacuum tins. R.W. Hills, a passionate innovator, developed a process that removed air from coffee packaging, resulting in fresher beans. Known as vacuum packing, this discovery has become the most used method to package coffee to this day. Unfortunately, for other roasters it was all-downhill from there. Soon local shops and mills around the country were all but extinguished by this new method of packaging. High Technology really was on the move; not only was the escalator invented the same year, so was instant coffee! Japanese-American chemist Satori Kato created a soluble blend of coffee and premiered it at the Pan-American Exposition. Every American was, and still is, in a rush. Rush. Rush. Everything must be instant. Who has time anymore? Maybe the Germans...

Those Germans, so fond of lingering over afternoon coffee, coined the term "Kaffee Klatsch" to describe women who gathered to converse of the day's latest views and gossip. Also around this time Ludwig Roselius, a German coffee importer and his assistant Karl Wimmer discovered a process to remove caffeine from the beans without wrecking the flavor of the coffee. The decaf discovery actually came about as the result of an accident. Coffee beans from Nicaragua had become water soaked during shipment. When the "ruined" beans arrived at Roselius' coffee warehouse, his researchers determined that the exposure to water had extracted much of the caffeine without affecting the taste, except for some saltiness. Not so fast, salty coffee? Yuck! Back-to-the-drawing-board! Soon they figured it out. The decaf process that Roselius and Wimmer invented used steam and chemical solvents. A later Swiss process would only use water. The brand name for this coffee would later become "Sanka" and made its way slowly to the U.S. some 20 years later.

The 1900s were a busy time in coffee history, at the beginning of the century an Italian, Luigi Bezzera, patented the first commercial "espresso" machine. The Tipo Gigante, was just that, a large steam driven machine that used a water and steam combination, forced under high pressure to brew the coffee at a rapid pace. His invention became known as the "espresso" machine. Legend has it; the initial reason for Luigi creating the espresso machine was to reduce the 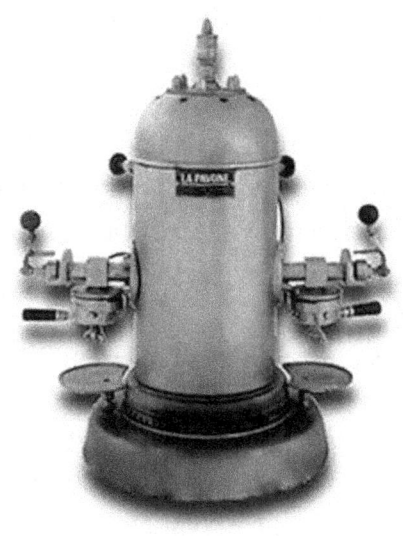 amount of time that his employees spent on their coffee break. Quite a taskmaster! Luigi needed them to work faster. So he thought that having a much quicker coffee maker would be the key to making employees spend less time on coffee breaks and more time working. "Productivity leads to profits," they say!

In 1908, Looking for a way to brew the perfect cup of coffee and remove those pesky grinds from floating around inside her cup, innovative German housewife Melitta Bentz created a coffee filter by using her son's school blotting paper. Mama knows best! A patent was awarded later that year and the Melitta Bentz Company was born. Oh, and remember that handsome Brazilian, Colonel Francisco de Melo Palheta who seduced and wooed the French Governor's wife -- all for Coffee? The daring tryst truly paid off: In this year, Brazil boasted 97% of the world's harvest. She truly did give away the farm back in 1727.

One of the pivotal events of the early 20th century was the First World War, also called the "War to end all wars", and the "War for Democracy", coffee played a part here too. The outbreak of World War I resulted in an immediate interruption of transatlantic trade. The European coffee exchanges closed. In countries involved in the war, stocks of coffee were impounded; the Brazilian coffee that was stored in Hamburg was bought up by the German government. In Britain, the Trading with the Enemy Act of the 18th of September 1914, forced all commercial banks in the City of London to break off business relations with the Central Powers. The British naval blockade prevented any goods in transit from being landed, and from November 1914 the British threatened to seize all the Central Powers' trading ships in the Mediterranean. These ships were to be held in harbor until the end of the war. Europe was largely cut off from the coffee-producing countries. While considerable stocks were held, it soon became apparent that the war would last longer than expected and that coffee would run out. The coffee-producing countries of South America, especially Brazil, experienced a deep slump in their foreign trade. The cultivation of coffee also experienced a crisis due to the lack of European investments.

The Central Powers could only buy coffee via neutral countries, mainly the Scandinavian countries and Holland. In 1915, Imperial Germany imported so much coffee from Brazil via Sweden that Brazil's coffee exports to Sweden jumped tenfold. Britain responded by imposing a ban on exports to the European continent on Sweden. Holland, under pressure from the British government, supplied the

Central Powers only with coffee from its own colonies. However, the robusta coffee produced in Holland's Asian colonies was not to continental tastes, and Britain increasingly pressured Holland to end all business with Central Powers. The Netherlands finally had to bow to British demands, although small amounts of coffee still entered Germany until March 1917. In the meantime, the South American coffee-producing countries had been able to resume production with the aid of US investments. The United States was now also the principal buyer of coffee beans. Increasing dependence on the USA meant that from 1917 the businesses of German-born producers and exporters in Latin America were expropriated and most of these countries, following the US, also entered the war.

In all belligerent countries, the import, distribution, and drinking of coffee was subjected to state or military control. Largely because of its attempt to control buying prices, Imperial Germany quickly became involved in the coffee trade through the *Zentrale Einkaufsgemeinschaft* (ZEG), a central buying association, but otherwise the trade remained free and in private hands. It was only with the beginning of the "total" phase of the war and the sharp decline in import options from 1916 onwards that the German government took over the entire coffee trade at all levels: import, wholesale, roasting, and retail. On 5 April 1916, the War Committee for Coffee, Tea, and Substitutes (*Kriegsausschuss für Kaffee, Tee und deren Ersatzstoffe*, KA) was set up. The KA formally took possession of all existing stocks of coffee and used them mainly to supply the army and the navy. A small amount was reserved to supply private consumers via the wholesale trade. Even black market coffee sources soon dried up. Unlike Germany and Austria, Britain and France were able to import significant amounts of coffee until the submarine war started and the USA entered the war in 1917. The British government tried to combine the coffee trade with its war aims to increase the amount of cargo space at its disposal when it offered to buy coffee from Brazil worth up to 3 million pounds sterling, if Brazil would hand over the forty-two German trading ships that were laid up in its harbors. Brazil refused, saying it was a "dirty deal" but later concluded a very similar deal with France.

Consumers in Imperial Germany and the Habsburg Empire, by contrast, largely had to do without coffee during the second half of the war, given that most of the ever-dwindling stocks of real coffee were made available to the army and the navy, leaving private consumers to make do with coffee substitutes. The poorer classes had mostly, but not exclusively, drunk substitutes before the war. Real coffee was drunk on Sundays and holidays, and was offered to important visitors, while for everyday consumption real coffee was mixed in with substitutes, most commonly, grains and chicory, crushed and roasted, to provide at least a trace of the real flavor. But from 1917 on even these products were rationed, and could only be obtained with a coffee ration card. In the final year of the war, a total ban was issued on roasting these substitutes, as grain for bread and chicory for animal feed took priority.

The collapse of the coffee trade as a consequence of the First World War had a long-term global and national impact. The USA was the only country to emerge strengthened from the war in this respect, as the collapse of the European markets allowed it to establish a dominant position in the coffee-producing countries of South America, as both an investor and as a buyer. The European market remained weak for many years to come, especially in Germany, which had been the most important European customer for coffee before 1914. The war was followed by a long period of state intervention in foreign trade, which hit coffee as a 'non-essential foodstuffs' particularly hard. The fact that the export, import, and consumption of coffee increased again after only a few years, and that this led to further crises of overproduction resulting in large-scale destruction of crops in Brazil, points to another lesson learned from the war. One of the things the German government in particular was measured by was whether it could keep the people adequately supplied with coffee. The time without coffee was long associated with WWI, but then also with the WWII, while the availability of coffee came to epitomize normality.

Come the dawn of the late 1930s as Adolf Hitler set his eyes on invading Poland, an action that led to the Second World War, the Brazilians were growing so much coffee and finding themselves with such a massive surplus, that their government approached Nestle in order to find a way to utilize the waste that ensues. Coffee guru, Max Morgenthaler, and his team set out to find a way of producing a quality cup of coffee that could be made simply by adding water, yet would retain the coffee's natural flavor. After seven long years of research and tinkering in their Swiss laboratories, (not very instant, mind you) they found their answer: "Waste not -- want not." Freeze dried coffee! No wonder the Swiss live in one of the richest and "greenest" countries in the world. The coffee was marketed as Nescafe and introduced in Switzerland. To this day, Nescafe is the world's leading brand.

By 1940 all of Europe was fighting another World War, Hitler and his axis powers were hellbent on conquest. And in yet another war, coffee would have a role to play as coffee was quickly rationed by both sides of WWII; they remembered the problem from the first war and acted quickly this time around. By this time, the governments of the world understood just how important coffee was to their fighting men and so established rationing on the home front to allow the combat troops to have a supply, albeit small, of everyone's favorite eye opener.

We are about to talk about the rationing of coffee in the United States during WWII, so let me ask you a simple question - "How much coffee do you drink? Could you get by with half as much?" That's what American civilians had to do during the months of U.S. coffee rationing in the Second World War.

During World War II, despite record coffee production in Brazil and other Latin American countries, the coffee supply in the U.S. was dwindling rapidly. This was obviously as a result of the war. Shipping was limited: all available ships were being diverted to the war effort the demands of the military on shipping space required diversion from importing coffee, and German U-boats were patrolling the shipping lanes and sinking merchant ships. To make sure men in uniform received enough, civilians had to do with less. In April 1942, the U.S. government limited coffee roasters to 75% of the previous year's supply. In September, the quota was cut to 65%. Finally, the Office of Price Administration found it necessary to ration coffee for civilians beginning November 29, 1942.

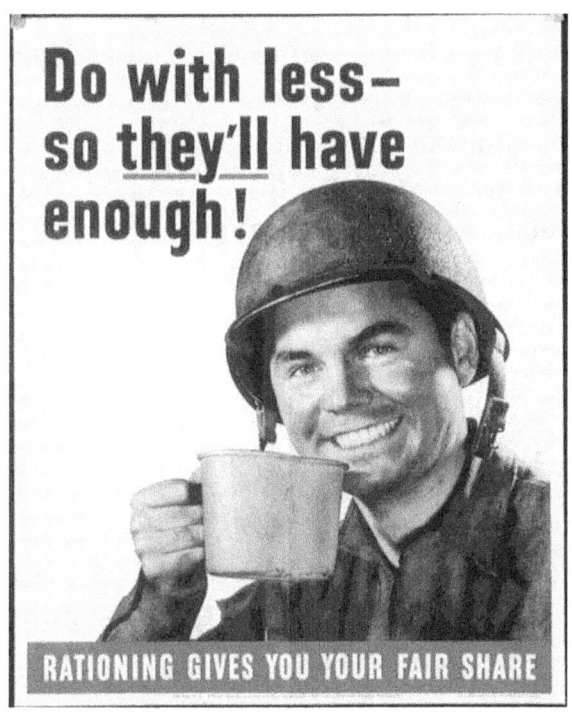

Mandatory coffee rationing made coffee available to all citizens on an equal basis, while giving priority to the needs of the military. Before the war, Americans were drinking more coffee than ever before. By this time, Coffee consumption in the United States had reached about 20 pounds for every American adult.

In 1940, the Ink Spots had a popular hit song called, "Java Jive." From September 1941 to April 1942, First Lady Eleanor Roosevelt had a popular weekly radio show called "Over Our Coffee Cups," which was sponsored by the Pan American Coffee Bureau. Coffee drinking was a way of life in the United States.

The wartime rationing regulations cut the amount of available coffee to just about half of what people had been used to. The initial rules allotted one pound of coffee every five weeks, or about ten pounds a year. Rationing was an important part of life in the United States during World War II. Although not necessary for survival, though that is debatable, coffee had been a staple in the American diet since the Boston Tea Party, and coffee rationing was extremely unpopular.

In preparation for rationing, in October 1942, sales of coffee were halted to prevent hoarding. On November 29, 1942, rationing began. Americans had already received War Ration Book One in May 1942 for sugar rationing, so the Office of Price Administration merely adjusted the value of the stamps. Stamps #19-28 were each designated for one pound of coffee during a specified five-week period. When the period expired, so did the stamp. Coffee stamps could only be redeemed for family members over the age of fifteen.

One pound every five weeks produced less than one cup per day. While some coffee drinkers benefitted from the generosity of non-coffee drinking friends or family members, most patriotic Americans made do with less. An article in the November 30th issue of Life magazine noted that the reduced availability gave coffee drinkers a choice: either they could drink about half as much good coffee as before, or they could "stretch" their coffee and continue drinking about the same amount.

The article went on to suggest various ways of stretching the coffee. It advised using a level, not heaping, tablespoon of coffee per cup, or adding chicory. To increase the yield, you could boil the coffee on the stove or use a percolator - People found if they used a bit less and percolated longer, they could stretch their ration a bit further. You could "double-drip" with a drip coffee maker (although the article acknowledged that coffee experts "frowned on" double dripping). When serving coffee, the article suggested filling the cup part way instead of to the brim. Reusing grounds made a watery beverage dubbed "Roosevelt coffee" in honor of the president.

Coffee substitutes such as chicory or Postum (wheat bran, wheat, molasses, and maltodextrin) were used grudgingly or mixed with real coffee. Another war victim was the familiar coffee can. Due to a shortage of tin, manufacturers packaged coffee in glass jars. Coffee shops that formerly offered a "bottomless cup" were now forced to limit a customer to a single cup. One coffee shop featured in the *Life* article did offer a second cup, but at a price of $100! (That was 1942 dollars – that is about $1480.69 in 2017 dollars!) The article doesn't say whether anyone accepted that offer.

Although Americans were very supportive of the war effort and the many sacrifices it entailed, we love our java and you can bet that coffee rationing was very unpopular. On February 3rd, 1943, the Office of Price Administration further reduced the coffee ration, allowing each person one pound every six weeks instead of five. In order to preserve supplies, consumers were also asked to spread out their coffee purchases over the six-week period instead of obtaining their entire ration at the beginning. On July 28th, 1943, President Roosevelt, who had patriotically switched his morning beverage from coffee to milk, announced the end of coffee rationing. Coffee was the first item to come off rationing. However, in September

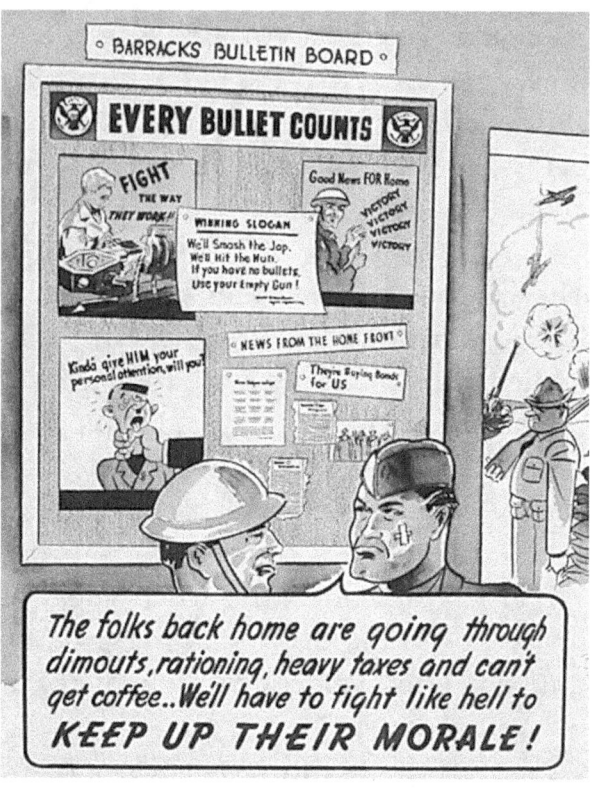

1944, the Office of Price Administration raised the price of coffee to curtail demand—under the threat of a return to rationing.

After WWII and on into the present-day coffee remained a strong and growing part of the American culture. In 1946, Achille Gaggia, evolved the espresso machine using a piston to extract the brew at a higher pressure resulting in a layer of "crema" on the coffee. Crema! OMG! The ultimate Espresso! The Cappuccino is born! One of the greatest discoveries of all time! Count your blessings the next time you order a double cappuccino for its named after the color and the likeness of the robes and hood of the Capuchin order of Franciscan Monks in Italy. Thank you, Achille Gaggia for delivering us this little bit of heaven-sent "crema" in a cup!

Coffee houses were, and are, still around and were, and are, still evolving with the times. In 1956 a modern generation of coffee houses took hold, not only pulsating to the new beat rhythms of Jazz, they also pulsated to the revolutionary avant-garde thoughts of the Beat Movement. As throughout history, once again coffee houses were central to debate, as well as the epicenter for cultural movements that defied the convention of the day. The more things change the more they stay the same, I suppose. At coffee shops in San Francisco's North Beach and in New York's Greenwich Village, the poets and intellectuals, known as Beatniks hung- out, drank espresso and had lively philosophical and political discussions that challenged the traditional ways of the 1950's. Beatniks and coffee houses go together - well, like beatniks and coffee houses!

These Bohemians were the forerunners of the cultural, political and sexual revolutions to come in the 1960's that were to change our world forever. Still to this day, these historic shops, as well as their counter-culture-counter-parts throughout the United States attract modern-day freethinkers who come together over a cup of coffee to share a bit of poetry, or discuss current events and generally move our societies forward. The dawn of the 1960s was huge in coffee history as The Colombian Coffee Federation that represents 560,000 coffee growers debuted the fictional spokesperson Juan Valdez, the humble Columbian coffee grower, who along with his loaded pack mule picks his beans one at a time.

Also In the 1960s, Alfred Peet, a Dutch-American, whose father ran a small roastery in Holland brought a little of the old country to his new country. In 1966, Alfred opened Peet's Coffee in Berkeley, California. He later is credited as the "grandfather" of the specialty coffee industry. Peet's is especially known for its strong, deep roasted coffee. His outstanding coffee would impact the world...

however as we will discover, it's a small world after all, smaller than you may know...

Peet's business flourished and by 1971, Alfred Peet shared and taught his style of roasting beans to three buddies, Jerry Baldwin, an english teacher, Zev Siegl a history teacher and Gordon Bowker, a writer. They worked over Christmas at the first Peet's store in Berkeley to learn the ropes. With Alfred's blessing, and his roasted beans, not only did they copy his store design, but they took his technique of roasting coffee beans and opened the first Starbucks in Seattle. Within a year, they acquired their own roaster and started roasting their own coffee. This store sold simply one thing: Fresh roasted coffee beans. That's it. Nothing else, no brewed drinks, no lattes, no snacks. Just fresh roasted coffee beans.

1972 saw a ground-breaking moment in coffee history as the first automatic drip coffee maker for home use was introduced. With the rather formal name of Mr. Coffee, it was introduced by Cleveland, Ohio entrepreneur Vincent Marotta. Please to meet you, Mr. Coffee. The innovation: water is percolated through the coffee grounds at 200° Fahrenheit, as opposed to the boiling water that roiled through grounds in the traditional percolator. Mr. Coffee was soon to become a household name because it was pitched on TV by the legendary baseball great and Hall of Fame recipient Joe DiMaggio maybe that success was a given. In the late 1970's 40,000 units each and every day were sold. It is still the world's best-selling coffee maker for home use. I own several.

As the 1980s rolled around the ground work was set for another milestone in coffee history, so let's get back to Starbucks. A major turning point is about to happen. A drip coffee maker salesman from New York spent a full year convincing the guys at Starbucks to hire him. He finally succeeded. Howard Schultz was hired and joined the team of Starbucks as their Director of Marketing. He set off to Milan, Italy where he saw cafés on practically every block. Places where one could have an outstanding espresso. These cafés also served as meeting places and he could see that they were a big part of the societal fabric. There were some 200,000 of them in Italy.

Back in Seattle, Schultz advised the company, they should sell coffee and espresso drinks, as well as the fresh roasted coffee beans they were becoming famous for. The owners Jerry, Zev, and Gordon rejected this idea outright, believing that getting into the beverage and restaurant business would distract the company from its primary focus. They believed 100% that fresh coffee should be brewed at home with their fresh roasted beans. No espressos or lattes would be made or served in their shops.

The original owners of Starbucks, led by Jerry Baldwin, purchased their mentor's business, Peet's In Seattle in 1984. Still believing very strongly in his café ideas, Howard Schultz certain that there was money to be made selling coffee drinks quit Starbucks and started the Il Giornale coffee chain in 1985. It was hugely successful.

By 1987 Schultz made an offer that the Starbucks ownership could not refuse. Eventually they gave in and Schultz bought Starbucks for a paltry $3.8 million. He finally secured their 'secret roasting techniques', rapidly renamed his own coffee chain "Starbucks" and changed forever how the world would buy their coffee beverages. It also changed how many books were written, much of this book was in fact penned at my local Starbucks while I indulged in a croissant and Caramel Macchiato. Schulz's big plan was now set in motion and his juggernaut steamed full-speed ahead!

In the 1990's, Starbucks opened a new store every workday, a pace that continued into the 2000's. one comedian of the time noted these coffee houses were opening so quickly that a new Starbucks just opened up in the Starbucks in his neighbourhood! Schultz left the CEO's leather backed chair and ascended to the throne of Chairman. He set out on his conquest of the world with a Starbucks in every country, on every corner, putting the Mom & Pop cafés out of business, and along the way gobbling up local café chains and renaming them as his own. After eight years of Starbucks rapid expansionist plans, in 2008 Schultz reclaimed the CEO position in order to bring back and restore what he called the "distinctive Starbucks experience" -- back to the core, back to basics... No more pre-ground coffee in the stores, only whole bean -- ground fresh once again. Catch me my friends, I think I am about to faint. Ground fresh? Imagine that? Others copied Schulz's idea but Starbucks is still the specialty coffee house leader. Specialty coffee now accounts for over 40% of all coffee sold in the United States. Hip-hip Hooray! Fresh roasted coffee! Fresh roasted coffee!

As we enter the new millennium the love of coffee remains strong. Today, coffee is the world's most popular beverage, bar none! We consume 400 billion cups each year, nearly 400 million cups a day. Why, I alone guzzle over 16,000 cups annually. The United States imports 27% of all coffee beans grown in the world. Coffee is second only to oil as the most traded commodity. So, let us pay homage and give credit where credit is due. So, as I say in the dedication to this book, let us raise our demitasse cups, our favorite old mugs, and our commuter cups to toast the thieves and smugglers to whom we truly owe our gratitude. Those unsung and unsavory heroes set forth the proliferation of coffee throughout the world and the variety of species we cherish today. Let us thank those through the centuries who toiled, battled, tinkered and seduced, all for that delectable cup of coffee, and for all of those who brought us to this wonderful place in coffee history, here's to you!

Thank you to all those farmers around the world who carefully nurture these cherries to fruition, the sourcers who travel to bring us these gifts, the artisan roasters who, with passion, finesse the roast of these beans to their ultimate degree, and thank you to all the baristas who brew us, each and every day, the wonderful cup we enjoy to our heart's content!

Let us all do our very best, make history everyday... with every sip we take.

7. Coffee as Medicine!

"Let food be thy medicine and medicine be thy food." This quote is attributed to Hippocrates. Another of my favorite quotes is *"Who said anything about medicine? Let's eat!"* which is attributed to one of Hippocrates forgotten (and hilarious) students. The same can be said for the drinks we consume – like coffee.

Who hasn't seen or heard Hippocrates' famous quote above? If you have Facebook friends who are the least bit into "natural" medicine or living, you've almost certainly come across it in your feed, and if you're a reader of my Phytonutrient Blog, you will absolutely have heard the quote. Now Hippocrates lived a very long time ago, that is definitely true but just because an idea is old, doesn't mean it's good, any more than just because Hippocrates said it means it must be true. But in this case, it does and it is!

Remember, Hippocrates was an important figure in the history of medicine because he was among the earliest to assert that diseases were caused by natural processes rather than the gods and because of his emphasis on the careful observation and documentation of patient history and physical findings, which led to the discovery of physical signs associated with diseases of specific organs. He is also known to have been a great healer because of his knowledge of the culinary and medicinal uses of herbs and spices. But you know what? Hippocrates was not the only advocate for letting food be thy medicine. Throughout the ages there have been many others. Ever since man first climbed down from the trees (or, depending upon your view, plucked that apple off that tree), eating has never been far from his 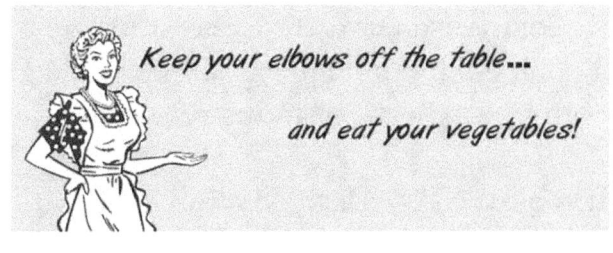 mind (survival has a way of prioritizing everything). The simple fact that sustenance equals life, means that food and health have culturally ridden shotgun throughout the ages.

"Good men eat and drink so they can live," noted Socrates.
"Eat, drink, and be merry!" commanded Solomon.
"You're famished. I'll fix you a plate!!" pleaded my mother.

In the days before medicine, food and drink was medicine…or at least it was seen as such. A browned apple for an upset stomach, chicken soup for congestion, champagne for septicemia (Pulitzer Prize-winning novelist Eudora Welty said her Mississippi father swore his use of the bubbly saved her ill mother's life). It was sometimes hard to establish cause and effect (Garlic as an anti-vampiric? Hard to find test subjects for that one,) and yet generations of pantries held foods sworn to bind, purge, ameliorate, instigate, invigorate…in short, improve one's well-being. And then came modern allopathic-oriented science, which until recently tossed nutrition—and its potential effect on both maintaining health and calming illness—into the compost heap. The reasons were myriad. Politically, no one had ever been elected on an anti-cheeseburger platform, so administrative pressure to funnel government dollars toward nutritional research traditionally was nil. Similarly, big pharma was scarce with cash, because they can't patent a food's natural properties. And from a practical viewpoint, studying food with its thousands of chemicals and nutrients is incredibly complex.

By comparison, targeting and studying a single drug for efficacy in a double-blind model was far more straightforward and lucrative to both researchers and industry.

It took the American Medical Association until 2002 to reverse a long-standing position and suggest that adults take a multivitamin every day. Then again, many of its long-standing members had never been exposed to a nutrition elective while in medical school...creating a drug-oriented bias that historically expressed itself in both the clinic and the lab.

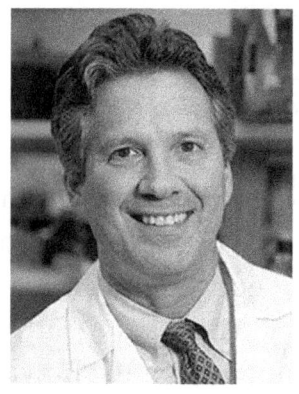

"I think for a long time the major directions in molecular biology—the ability to make genetically altered mice that could measure the impacts of certain molecules on the body—was totally not applied to nutrition," - Hopkins' William Nelson, director of the Sidney Kimmel Cancer Center.

That Nelson can speak of such research deficiencies in the past tense is indicative of a huge shift toward nutritional research in just the past 10 to 15 years. Again, I remind you that the information I present in this series, while in truth very old is now being backed by 21st Century science and research!

What then is the catalyst for this paradigm shift in thinking? Well since you asked I'll tell you what I think. We can't seem to shut our mouths, and the stats from the Centers for Disease Control back that up! With the exception of Colorado dwellers, more than 20% of the U.S. population is now considered obese. Given obesity's epidemiologically supported impact on cardiac, vascular, cancer, and diabetic-related illness, researchers are now branching out to uncover the myriad ways food and its micro components enhance or disrupt life. The sheer numbers of nutritional studies bear out this interest. According to Pub Med, such published investigations more than doubled between the 1980s and 1990s, and leapt another 71% this decade. Part of the quantum leap in the last five years especially, is the discovery that chronic inflammation is slowly being linked to diseases including cancer, and that foods—from cloves to walnuts—appear to contain anti-inflammatory properties.

This critical mass of information even has a name. Called the 'Food as Medicine movement', it's a growing recognition on the part of many academic clinicians that to ignore the role of food and nutrition in health is to lose a valuable tool that can support (or perhaps even lessen or replace) many pharmaceuticals currently in use.

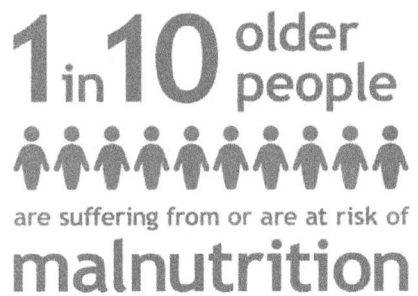

1 in 10 older people

are suffering from or are at risk of

malnutrition

"The perfect example is ginger," says Hopkins gastroenterologist Gerard Mullin, arguably the nation's top expert on the relationship between food and gut disorders. *"People who have nausea, or gastric dysmotilities or other GI problems, for them ginger is at the top of my list. It works the same way (the big pharma produced) Zofran does, which is one of our most powerful anti-nausea drugs. It works on the same receptor in the brain. But a lot of docs aren't aware of it."*

Similarly, food plays a huge role in how well people battle cancer. Researchers estimate that some 80% of cancer patients are malnourished, at the very time when chemotherapy often increases the body's need for proteins and other nutrients. Such malnourishment, if not addressed, can lead to a reduction of chemotherapy doses and ultimately poorer outcomes. Oncologist Bill Nelson says that the link between calories taken in—the so-called "caloric budget"—and its relationship to cancer is of great interest to him. Nelson notes that caloric intake drops among the elderly, while their cancer rates rise. It may well be that taking in fewer calories— especially of food of little to no nutritional value—leaves elders deprived of nutrients they need to stave off cancer, he says.

The thirst for nutritional knowledge is by no means limited to physicians and wellness professionals. A poll of attendees of <u>A Women's Journey</u>, an annual women's health symposium sponsored by Hopkins Medicine, showed a huge demand for more seminars devoted to the nuances of nutrition, and faculty speakers who could make sense of the flood of dietary data being unleashed on the public. In response, the Fall 2009 <u>A Woman's Journey</u> featured numerous talks with a nutritional component, including three seminars—led by the aforementioned Nelson, Mullin, and nutritionist Lynda McIntyre—that, like a well-balanced meal, triangulated how different research approaches are translating into smarter ways to eat for health. For Gerard Mullin, nutrition and health have always been intertwined. What's different now is the scientific rigor being applied to the field.

"My mom had the first health food store in northern New Jersey. I've cooked since I was 10," says Mullin. *"I was raised on food as medicine, and I'm glad the science has really borne out and supported what many of us were raised to believe since we were yay high."* Mullin refers to himself as an integrative gastroenterologist, the adjective referring to physicians who use complementary modalities including stress management and nutrition in their clinical practices. In both interviews and talks, Mullin lays out a compelling explanation for the mind/body connection to the gut, and

how different foods, spices, and herbs can promote better digestive health, especially in the 90 million Americans suffering from digestive diseases. He focuses on the common negative feedback loop affecting the "cephalic" phase of digestion—the gastric and saliva secretions that occur when appetite is stimulated but before eating actually begins. Sleep deprivation, emotional upset, poor eating habits—all can lead to an impaired cephalic phase. It's the stomach's equivalent of not being in the mood, and the response is somewhat the same. Diminished blood flow impairs function: In this case the gut doesn't absorb nutrients. All that unabsorbed food can make us miserable (i.e., everything from diarrhea to gas, bloating, and beyond). That jacks up stress levels, makes eating even more undesirable, and before you know it you've worked yourself into a case of irritable bowel syndrome or worse.

While drugs can treat symptoms, Mullin says breaking the cycle is both a mental and physical process. Taking the time to cook can in itself enhance that first cephalic phase—everything from the meditative act of chopping to inhaling rich aromas can be relaxing— while choosing certain foods such as peppermint leaves and ground flax may reduce gut spasms.

According to British Medical Journal studies, Mullin says, *"Peppermint works better than most IBS drugs. It works on relaxing calcium channel blockers. Sometimes it can* make your gut so relaxed, right between the gut and esophagus, that you get some burping or heartburn, so you have to be careful how much you use. More isn't always better."

1 in 3 people aged 65+ are at risk of malnutrition on admission to hospital

At Hopkins, Mullin has worked to improve both nutrition and timely access to food given to Johns Hopkins Hospital inpatients. *"In a hospital setting, anywhere from 33% to 55% of people are malnourished,"* he notes. With study funding from Department of Medicine Chief Mike Weisfeldt, says Mullin, "we proved that if you feed people earlier (following admission), their hospital stay is shorter and outcome is much better. It is common sense, but we had to show the evidence. And it's reawakened a whole discussion" about improving gut health through diet. Mullin notes that many common kitchen staples can be very effective for preventing and relieving gut-related maladies. *"Caraway has been well-studied,"* Mullin says. *"Its oil is a treatment for gastroparesis, so for those with slow motility and problems with their upper GI tract, caraway can promote motility. Fennel, ginger, dill, cumin...all these things can help you on an everyday basis."*

From both a taste and nutrient viewpoint, fresh is generally better than dried, though dried is better than nothing. As for amounts, most research suggests moderation as a key, the idea being that it's the continuous, sustainable addition of herbs and other nutrients that enhance flavor and long-term gut health. Do not skip meals, eating regularly and including herbs and spices, fruit and vegetables, and fish is truly necessary to optimum health especially in our young and elderly.

Equally important is what foods to avoid. Improving that cephalic response will be pretty much a waste if the gut is being overdosed with junk. Mullin cites studies noting that, while the average American consumes 100 grams of fructose a day—

22% of people aged 60+ **skipped meals** to cut back on **food costs**

everything from "soda to ketchup to grapes"—the body can only tolerate about 50 grams. The overload acts as an IBS and gas trigger. *"The first thing we do is say, 'Look, if you want to get better, you have to find a way to eliminate some of these sugars."* He says. Mullin aims his last culinary salvo at inflammation. Many scientists believe that certain aspects of lifestyle—notably what we eat—can create a chronic inflammatory state within cells, tissues, and organs. In short, the immune system is in constant attack mode, which may have deleterious effects on health. *"We know that many conditions in the gut are mediated through inflammation. We're appreciating that now more than ever,"* he says, pointing to recent research links. *"How do you help make yourself better? Again, it's a food as medicine approach. There are (anti-inflammatory) studies about blueberries and blackberries out there (see "Allies in the Pantry.")*

Bill Nelson's interest in food literally comes down to a flip of the wrist. No, not as a chef, but rather a scientist fascinated by how foods—notably meats—are altered by the way they're cooked. Using World Health Organization data, Nelson concluded that some 35% of cancers probably include a dietary element, with inflammation—which could also have dietary factors—playing a role in perhaps another 30% of cases. A highly respected molecular biologist and cancer clinician—he's principal investigator for one of the National Cancer Institute's Specialized Program of Research Excellence (SPORE) initiatives—Nelson has taken a microscopic interest in the interplay of diet and prostate cancer. He notes that not only do Asian men have far less prostate cancer than their American counterparts, they appear far less prone to inflammation. When comparing autopsies of non-cancerous prostates of men who live in America versus those in Asia, *"Every prostate removed here showed signs of inflammation, while the Asian prostates were pristine."* Curiously, the longer Asian men are in America, the more likely they are to develop prostate cancer. *"If they're here 25 years or more, their rate becomes half that of Caucasians, and if their kids are born here, their risk is the same as Caucasians. There must be something in the lifestyle risks that we can reduce."* While Asians tend to eat far more fish and far less meat and fowl than Americans, Nelson says that might not tell the whole story. The problem may lie in how we heat our meats. *"Heat changes a huge amount of the components in food,"* says Nelson, focusing on two particular carcinogens that can be created by cooking. The first, called heterocyclic amines, are formed by the heat-catalyzed interplay between creatinine (found in the muscle of meats and fish) and amino acids.

One heterocyclic amine called "PhIP" is extremely nasty: When given to rats in doses comparable to those consumed by humans, the male rats rapidly developed prostate and colon cancer, while the female rats developed colon and breast cancer.

"For us, that was fascinating," recalled Nelson. *"We just said, 'Holy cow! It is incredible that something you could eat could do that."*

37% of people aged **70+** who have recently moved into care homes are at risk of **malnutrition**

Not only can the amount and duration of heat increase these dangerous amines (i.e., well-done appears worse for you than medium or medium rare), but so can cooking technique. *"You can take burger patties, put them on the same skillet, control for temperature and time, but in one case you flip them only once, in the middle of cooking, while the other you flip every 30 seconds."* The burgers only flipped once *"make a ton of amines,"* notes Nelson. *"So did sausages cooked as links versus patties."* The links, in Nelson's opinion, act *"as closed reaction vessels.*" Nelson's own research uncovered that in many cases the liver can't metabolize all these "charred" meat carcinogens, and passes them through to the prostate, where people with a particular DNA mutation may be at much higher risk for developing cancer.

Nelson also points out that the fat dripping along a deep grilled steak might taste delicious, but it's potentially deadly. The culprit, which also escapes from the fat in chicken skin, is something called polycyclic aromatic hydrocarbon carcinogens. To put some numbers to the science, Nelson says the amount of these carcinogens consumed daily by the average American *"equals ingesting half a pack of cigarette smoke a day."*

My suggestion: **If you're going to eat meat, and I am, then stick to lower-fat cuts, take the skin off of chicken before cooking, and look at alternatives such as broiling or, in the case of fish, poaching the filet. Remember too that fat in the diet is important, but it is the right fats – like olive oil or the fats that are found in fish that we need – not a ton of beef or poultry fats.**

Nelson believes that both the public and industry are ready to hear his message. In meetings with executives at a large grocery store, Nelson discovered that 16% of the chain's sales came from pre-cooked foods and meals that busy customers quickly reheated at home. The executives had quite an appetite for Nelson's food prep science. Not only would such techniques improve food safety, but long term, the executives saw such preparatory expertise as potentially marketable to health-conscious consumers. *"I'm tantalized by the way we could affect broad-based cooking practices,"* he says *"We're at the dawn of an era of figuring this out."*

Figuring out how to translate serious science into tasty, healthy snacks and meals is where nutritionist Lynda McIntyre excels. A registered dietitian with a specialty counseling cancer patients at both the Kimmel Cancer Center at Hopkins and the Sibley Hospital Center for Breast Health in Washington D.C., McIntyre took A Woman's Journey attendees on a virtual tour of the supermarket. Along the way, she busted some myths regarding what it is about food that links it to perhaps the majority of cancer cases.

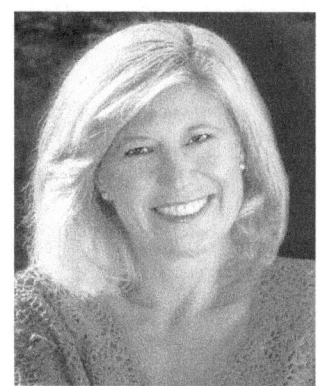

"A lot of times people think I'm talking about pesticides or additives in food, when in fact I'm not," she says. *"Less than 2% percent of all cancers can be directly related to what the additives are in food. Up to 60 percent can be related to what we're not eating."*

<u>Read that quote again</u> – I know that we are all concerned about pesticides in our food, as we should be, but we need to be at least equally concerned about what **we are and are not eating!** As in enough fruits and vegetables. A familiar message, yes, but McIntyre gives it a twist, suggesting shoppers take a colorful approach to solving their qualms about which produce has the greatest overall benefits. You have heard me say it and now this doctor stresses it too, *"Eat the rainbow. The brighter the food, the richer the color, the higher its anti-oxidant count,"* counsels McIntyre, who also served on a statewide council that developed cancer prevention strategies for Maryland. For McIntyre and other savvy nutritionists, the state of food science has allowed them to fine-tune their message and take some of the confusion out of the game. Take fresh versus frozen produce. McIntyre says both are effective…

"*Fresh is always best when it is in season,*" says McIntyre, since fresh produce retains top flavor and nutritional value. However, McIntyre notes that many fresh foods have relatively short seasons. As an alternative, from a nutritional viewpoint, "*frozen can be just as nutritious because it's picked at the peak of ripeness, and frozen to keep the nutritional content intact.*"

Then there's eating whole foods versus taking supplements, a source of huge debate. The prevailing sentiment among many researchers is that supplementation can bring someone deficient in a given nutrient up to a supportive baseline, but people already at solid baseline levels may not benefit from additional dosing.

93% of malnourished older people are in the community.

"*In some cases, single supplementation of antioxidants can increase the risk of certain diseases,*" says McIntyre. "*For example, vitamin E and heart disease. Another example is that single supplementation of vitamin A can increase bone fractures in women. And in smokers who took beta-carotene, we saw an increase in lung cancer. The studies show it is the whole foods (and how they work together synergistically) that provides the most protective effect to the body.*"

Knowing how to combine those foods can increase the body's ability to absorb their nutrients. McIntyre says putting broccoli (sulforaphane) and tomatoes (lycopene) together "*increases their tumor protective ability.*" Similarly, carrots and avocado are a nice dynamic duo because beta-carotene is better absorbed in the presence of a fat (short on avocados? Try olive oil). Apples and blueberries, even spinach and strawberries (*"It's a strange combination, but delicious,"* insists McIntyre) all make for nutrient-dense dynamic duos.

So, bottom line, what I want, and need, for you to understand is this; as for the thinking that healthy eating and drinking is restrictive, forget it. Nearly every family of food and beverage that I have researched—be it nut, fruit, spice, fish, grain, beans, chocolate, wine, beer or coffee, has some and very often many, members in it filled with high nutritional content, when we consume them in moderation. On every conceivable front, from the molecular level to the kitchen table, research is unlocking the power of certain foods and drinks to keep us in fighting shape. Since none of us has a "foodprint" yet—a DNA or some other molecular roadmap that will tell us why Sally's system can absorb beta-carotene from carrots, while Sue's can only assimilate that same beta-carotene from sweet potatoes—for now, eating a well-rounded, well-informed diet containing moderate amounts of a wide varieties of fresh foods and drinks, is all about playing the odds. And there's nothing better than improving your chances of beating the house.

So, the next time that someone tries to tell you that you shouldn't be drinking that Latte Macchiato – just tell them that they shouldn't worry, you are just working on improving your health!

8. Health Benefits of Coffee

When I was a kid, my parents refused to let me drink coffee because they believed it would "stunt my growth." It turns out, of course, that this is a myth. Studies have failed, again and again, to show that coffee or caffeine consumption are related to reduced bone mass or how tall people are or will grow to be.

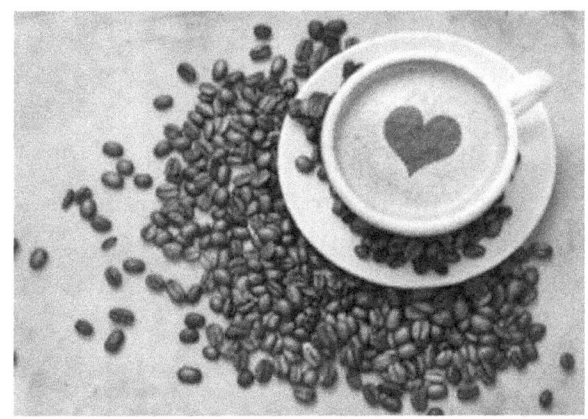

This just demonstrates that coffee has long had a reputation as being unhealthy. But in almost every single respect that reputation is backward. The potential health benefits of moderate coffee consumption are surprisingly large.

When I set out to look at the research on coffee and health, I thought I'd see it being associated with some good outcomes and some bad ones, mirroring the contradictory reports you can often find in the news media. This didn't turn out to be the case.

Just last year, a systematic review and meta-analysis of studies looking at long-term consumption of coffee and the risk of cardiovascular disease was published. The researchers found 36 studies involving more than 1,270,000 participants. The combined data showed that those who consumed a moderate amount of coffee, about three to five cups a day, were at the lowest risk for problems.

Those who consumed five or more cups a day had no higher risk than those who consumed none.

Of course, everything I'm saying here concerns coffee — black coffee. I am not talking about the mostly milk and sugar coffee-based beverages that lots of people consume. These could include, but aren't limited to, things like:

- McDonald's large mocha (500 calories, 17 grams of fat, 72 grams of carbohydrates)
- Starbucks Venti White Chocolate Mocha (580 calories, 22 grams of fat, 79 grams of carbs)
- Large Dunkin' Donuts frozen caramel coffee Coolatta (670 calories, 8 grams of fat, 144 grams of carbs)
- Cold Stone Creamery Gotta-Have-It-Sized Lotta Caramel Latte (1,790 calories, 90 grams of fat, 223 grams of carbs)

Regular brewed coffee has 5 or fewer calories and no fat or carbohydrates.

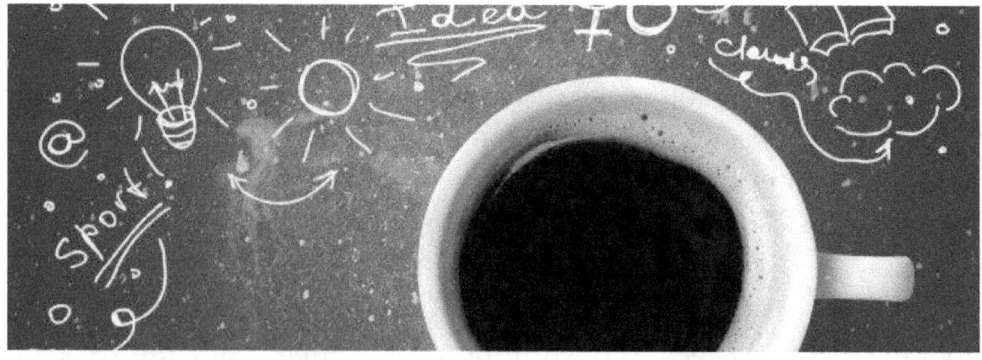

Back to the studies. Years earlier, a meta-analysis, which by the way, means a study of studies, in which data are pooled and analyzed together, was published looking at how coffee consumption might be associated with stroke. Eleven studies were found, including almost 480,000 participants. As with the prior studies, consumption of two to six cups of coffee a day was associated with a lower risk of disease, compared with those who drank none. Another meta-analysis published a year later confirmed these findings.

Rounding out concerns about the effect of coffee on your heart, another meta-analysis examined how drinking coffee might be associated with heart failure. Again, moderate consumption was associated with a lower risk, with the lowest risk among those who consumed four servings a day. Consumption had to get up to about 10 cups a day before any bad associations were seen.

No one is suggesting you drink more coffee for your health. But drinking moderate amounts of coffee is linked to lower rates of pretty much all cardiovascular disease, contrary to what many might have heard about the dangers of coffee or caffeine. Even consumers on the very high end of the spectrum appear to have minimal, if any, ill effects. This is not my speculation here, this is a thoroughly researched and proven fact.

But let's not cherry-pick. There are outcomes outside of heart health that matter. Many believe that coffee might be associated with an increased risk of cancer. Certainly, individual studies have found that to be the case, and these are sometimes highlighted by the news media. But taken all together, most of these negative outcomes disappear.

A meta-analysis published in 2007 found that increasing coffee consumption by two cups a day was associated with a lower relative risk of liver cancer by more than 40 percent. Two more recent studies confirmed these findings. Results from meta-analyses looking at prostate cancer found that in the higher-quality studies, coffee consumption was not associated with negative outcomes.

The same holds true for breast cancer, where associations were statistically not significant. It's true that the data on lung cancer shows an increased risk for more coffee consumed, but that's only among people who smoke. Drinking coffee may be protective in those who don't. Regardless, the authors of that study hedge their results and warn that they should be interpreted with caution because of the confounding (and most likely overwhelming) effects of smoking. A study looking at all cancers suggested that it might be associated with reduced overall cancer incidence and that the more you drank, the more protection was seen.

Drinking coffee is associated with better laboratory values in those at risk for liver disease. In patients who already have liver disease, it's associated with a decreased progression to cirrhosis. In patients who already have cirrhosis, it's associated with a lower risk of death and a lower risk of developing liver cancer. It's associated with improved responses to antiviral therapy in patients with hepatitis C and better outcomes in patients with nonalcoholic fatty liver disease. The authors of the systematic review argue that daily coffee consumption should be encouraged in patients with chronic liver disease.

The most recent meta-analyses on neurological disorders found that coffee intake was associated with lower risks of Parkinson's disease, lower cognitive decline and a potential protective effect against Alzheimer's disease (but certainly no harm).

A systematic review published in 2005 found that regular coffee consumption was associated with a significantly reduced risk of developing Type 2 diabetes, with the lowest relative risks (about a third reduction) seen in those who drank at least six or seven cups a day. The latest study, published in 2014, used updated data and included 28 studies and more than 1.1 million participants. Again, the more coffee you drank, the less likely you were to have diabetes. This included both caffeinated and decaffeinated coffee.

Is coffee associated with the risk of death from all causes? There have been two meta-analyses published within the last year or so. The first reviewed 20 studies, including almost a million people, and the second included 17 studies containing more than a million people. Both found that drinking coffee was associated with a significantly reduced chance of death. I can't think of any other product that has this much positive epidemiologic evidence going for it.

I grant you that pretty much none of the research I'm citing above contains randomized controlled trials. It's important to remember that we usually see those trials conducted to see if what we are observing in epidemiologic studies holds up. Most of us aren't drinking coffee because we think it will protect us, though. Most of us are worrying that it might be hurting us. There's almost no evidence for that at all.

If any other modifiable risk factor had these kinds of positive associations across the board, the media would be all over it. Doctors would be pushing it on everyone. Whole interventions would be built up around it. For far too long, though, coffee has been considered a vice, not something that might actually be healthy.

That may change soon. The newest scientific report for the U.S.D.A. nutritional guidelines, which I've discussed before, says that coffee is not only O.K. — it agrees that it might be good for you. This was the first time the dietary guideline advisory committee reviewed the effects of coffee on health.

There's always a danger in going too far in the other direction. I'm not suggesting that we start serving coffee to little kids. Caffeine still has a number of effects parents might want to avoid for their children. Some people don't like the way caffeine can make them jittery. Guidelines also suggest that pregnant women not drink more than two cups a day.

I'm also not suggesting that people start drinking coffee by the gallon. I cannot say enough that moderation is the key to good health! Too much of anything can be bad. Finally, while the coffee may be healthy, that's not necessarily true of the added sugar and fat that many people put into coffee-based beverages.

But it's way past time that we stopped viewing coffee as something we all need to cut back on. It's a completely reasonable addition to a healthy diet, with more potential benefits seen in research than almost any other beverage we're consuming. It's time we started treating it as such. So, understand that there are good reasons to drink coffee and sure, there are a few reasons not to. This book is written by a big-time coffee proponent and is intended for those that are looking for reasons to keep drinking their morning brew. After all, you may have a caffeine-hater in your life. You know the type, they're always telling you what's bad for your health.

Here's a list of some good reasons to drink coffee. Memorize this list, that way, the next time you encounter your favorite coffee-hater you can pull out one of these babies. While you're at it, you can add the words *"from a peer-reviewed scientific journal"* — that'll really get your pet coffee-hater frothing at the mouth!

Cut the Pain

Two cups of coffee can cut post-workout muscle pain by up to 48%. *From the Journal of Pain, March 2007*

Increase your fiber intake

A cup of brewed coffee represents a contribution of up to 1.8 grams of fiber of the recommended intake of 20-38 grams. *From the Journal of Agricultural and Food Chemistry*

Protection against cirrhosis of the liver

Of course, you could just cut down on the alcohol intake. *From the Archives of Internal Medicine.* Another more recent study also showed coffee's liver protecting benefits. Yet another study showed that both coffee and decaffeinated coffee lowered the liver enzyme levels of coffee drinkers. This study was published in the Hepatology Journal.

Lowered risk of Type 2 Diabetes

Those who consumed 6 or more cups per day had a 22% lower risk of diabetes. *From the Archives of Internal Medicine.* A recent review of research conducted by Harvard's Dr. Frank Hu showed that the risk of type II diabetes decreases by 9% for each daily cup of coffee consumed. Decaf coffee decreased risk by 6% per cup.

Lowered risk of Alzheimer's disease

There is considerable evidence that caffeine may protect against Alzheimer's disease. *From the European Journal of Neurology.*

Reduces suicide risk and Depression

A 10-year study of 86,000 female nurses shows a reduced risk of suicide in the coffee drinkers. *From the Archives of Internal Medicine.* Another study conducted by the Harvard School of Public Health found that women who drink 4 or more cups of coffee were 20% less likely to suffer from depression.

Protection against Parkinson's

People with Parkinson's disease are less likely to be smokers and coffee drinkers than their healthy siblings. Just make sure you don't get lung cancer on the way. *From the Archives of Neurology.* Even newer research out of Sweden revealed that drinking coffee reduces the risk of Parkinson's even when genetic factors come into play.

Coffee drinkers have less risk of heart disease.

Korean researchers found that study participants who consumed 3 to 5 cups of coffee a day were less likely to show the beginning signs of heart disease. *Other dietary factors should also be noted as Koreans typically have a different diet than do Westerners.*

Coffee drinkers have stronger DNA.

A study published in the European Journal of Nutrition showed that coffee drinkers have DNA with stronger integrity since the white blood cells of coffee drinkers had far less instance of spontaneous DNA strand breakage.

Lower Risk of Multiple Sclerosis.

Recent research showed that at least 4 cups of coffee a day may help protect against the development and reoccurrence of MS. It is believed that the coffee prevents the neural inflammation that possibly leads to the disease developing. The study was published in the *Journal of Neurology, Neurosurgery & Psychiatry.*

Coffee reduces colorectal cancer risk.

Even moderate consumption of coffee can reduce the odds of developing colorectal cancer by 26%. This protective benefit increases with more consumption.

Coffee is the biggest source of Antioxidants in the western diet

For people who eat a standard Western diet, coffee may actually be the healthiest aspect of the diet. That's because coffee contains a **massive** number of antioxidants. In fact, studies show that most people get more antioxidants from coffee than both fruits and vegetables… combined (We all need to eat more fruit and veg!)
2004 The American Society for Nutritional Sciences

Well there you go, there are a dozen good reasons to drink your coffee, but how about a few more just for the fun of it.

1. **Reduced Liver Cancer Risk:** Researchers at USC Norris Comprehensive Cancer Center found that those that consume 1-3 cups of coffee a day have a 29% reduced risk of developing liver cancer (hepatocellular carcinoma (HCC), which is the most common type.
2. **Less Gout Risk:** Yet another reason: Risk for developing gout (in men) decreases with increasing coffee consumption. This is a large study of over 50,000 men.
3. **Longevity:** Greek boiled coffee linked to longevity and heart health. Another study published in the June 17, 2008, issue of the *Annals of Internal Medicine* showed that women who consume coffee had a lower risk of death from cancer, heart disease, and other factors, which therefore promotes a longer lifespan. Yet another study published in the New England Journal of Medicine showed that coffee drinkers were at less risk of dying prematurely from diseases like diabetes, heart disease and forms of cancer. Another study from Japan found that men who drink at least 3 cups of coffee per day have a 24% less risk of dying early from disease. Yet another study from Harvard also confirmed that those who drink 1-5 cups of coffee a day avoid diseases linked to premature death.
4. **Prevents Retinal Damage**. A Cornell University Study showed that coffee may prevent retinal damage due to oxidative stress. Caffeine isn't the culprit here, but chlorogenic acid (CLA), which is one of the strong antioxidants found in the coffee bean.
5. **Black coffee prevents cavities**. Researchers out of Brazil found that strong black coffee kills the bacteria on teeth that leads to tooth decay. Adding milk or sugar to coffee negates this benefit.
6. **Coffee may protect against periodontal disease**. As part of the US Department of Veterans Affairs Dental Longitudinal

Study coffee consumption and dental health among 1,152 men was tracked from 1968-1998. The researchers found that coffee didn't promote gum disease and actually showed a protective benefit.

7. **Coffee may protect against melanoma**. A study published in the Journal of the National Cancer Institute found that melanoma risk decreases with coffee consumption and that this risk decreases with each cup consumed.

8. **The USDA's new 2015 dietary guidelines recommend it for better health**. They advise people that having 3 to 5 cups of coffee a day is good for their overall health and reduces the risk of disease. However, they report that adding sugar, cream, or flavored creamers quickly negates the potential benefits.

9. **Reduced heart attack mortality risk**. Researchers found that those who drink two or more cups of coffee daily after having a heart attack have the least risk of dying from the heart attack.

Conclusion

Look, while I could bow to convention and follow the "rules" of proper book layout and publishing, those that demand that in the conclusion I sum up all of the preceding chapters and answer any questions that may still remain in the minds of my readers, I would rather not.

Frankly I just don't want to do that. So, since I have never much been one for following all the "rules," I think I'll just approach this conclusion the way I want.

You see, I absolutely do not want to answer all of your questions with this book. In fact, I think that all of those so called, "all you need to know" books are ridiculous!

What I want to achieve with this work, what hope I have achieved is that I provided you with enough solid, scientific information that you are encouraged to start asking more questions about everything you consume; their history, their impact on mankind, and their possible impact on your health. I hope you do some additional research of your own!

As for how I would sum up this book? Let me simply paraphrase something I said many times earlier in this work…

Too much of a good thing is not a good thing! Ridiculously increased coffee consumption over time will not lead to better health but could, and usually will, in fact, ruin your health.

Moderation is the key word here!

I will leave you with just a few more bits of graphical information to consider. If nothing I have written in this book has got you thinking than maybe one of these will:

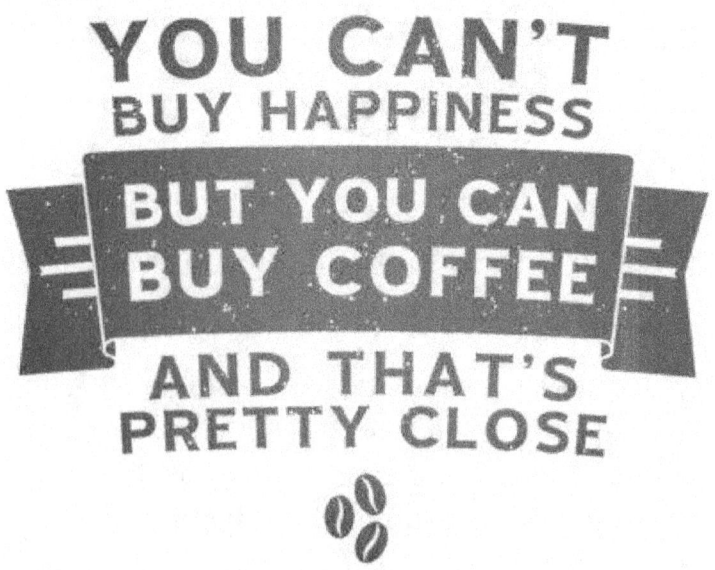

Health Benefits of
Drinking Coffee

Rich Source of
Antioxidants

Can Make You
Happy

May Decrease
STRESS

Can Improve
Energy Level

May Reduce
Pain

Can Prevent
Alzheimers

May Burn
Fat

Can Make You
Smarter

Great for Your
Liver

Can Reduce
Diabetes Risk

Keeps Brain
Healthy Longer

Can Reduce
Suicide Risk

T h e
Second
M o s t
Popular
D r i n k
In   The
World
A f t e r
Water

IT IS SO
YUMMY

Moderate amounts of caffeine can increase the size of the hippocampus which aids in short and long term memory.

Trigonelline is a compound found in coffee that contains anti-bacterial & anti-adhesive properties that help prevent tooth decay and cavities.

Coffee can reduce the risk of breast cancer in menopausal women, and it also fights the formation of colon cancer. The antioxidents in coffee can also help precent uterine & ovarian cancer.

Studies found that coffee intake lowers the level of a stress hormone in pregnant women.

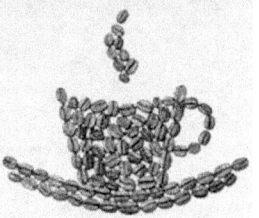

BENEFITS OF COFFEE

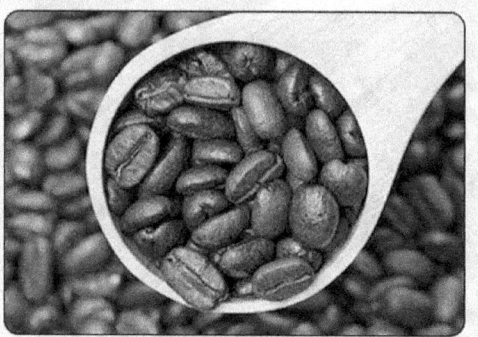

Aids in weight loss

Reduces risk of developing diabetes

Energizes and activates mind and body

Beneficial in preventing liver and colorectal cancer

Regular drinking prevents heart diseases

Protects liver against cirrhosis and hepatitis

Helps to regulate metabolic activity of body

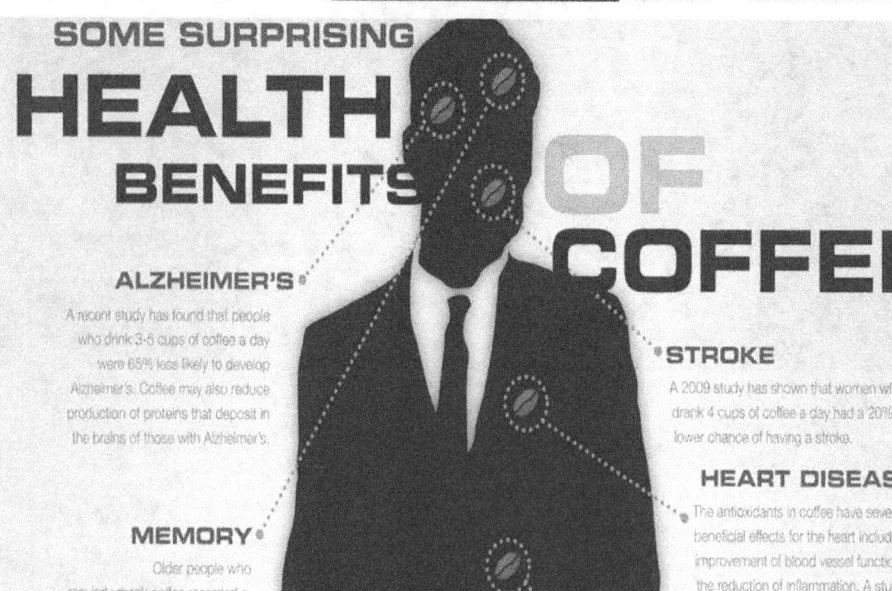

SOME SURPRISING HEALTH BENEFITS OF COFFEE

ALZHEIMER'S
A recent study has found that people who drink 3-5 cups of coffee a day were 65% less likely to develop Alzheimer's. Coffee may also reduce production of proteins that deposit in the brains of those with Alzheimer's.

MEMORY
Older people who regularly drank coffee recorded a slower rate of cognitive decline.

STROKE
A 2009 study has shown that women who drank 4 cups of coffee a day had a 20% lower chance of having a stroke.

HEART DISEASE
The antioxidants in coffee have several beneficial effects for the heart including the improvement of blood vessel function and the reduction of inflammation. A study has also shown that women who drink 2-3 cups a day have a 25% lower risk of death from heart disease.

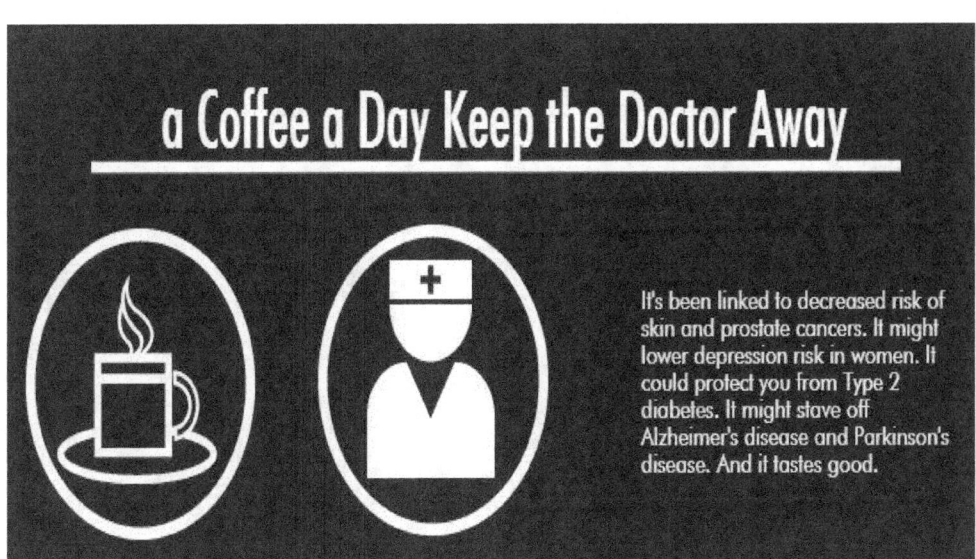

a Coffee a Day Keep the Doctor Away

It's been linked to decreased risk of skin and prostate cancers. It might lower depression risk in women. It could protect you from Type 2 diabetes. It might stave off Alzheimer's disease and Parkinson's disease. And it tastes good.

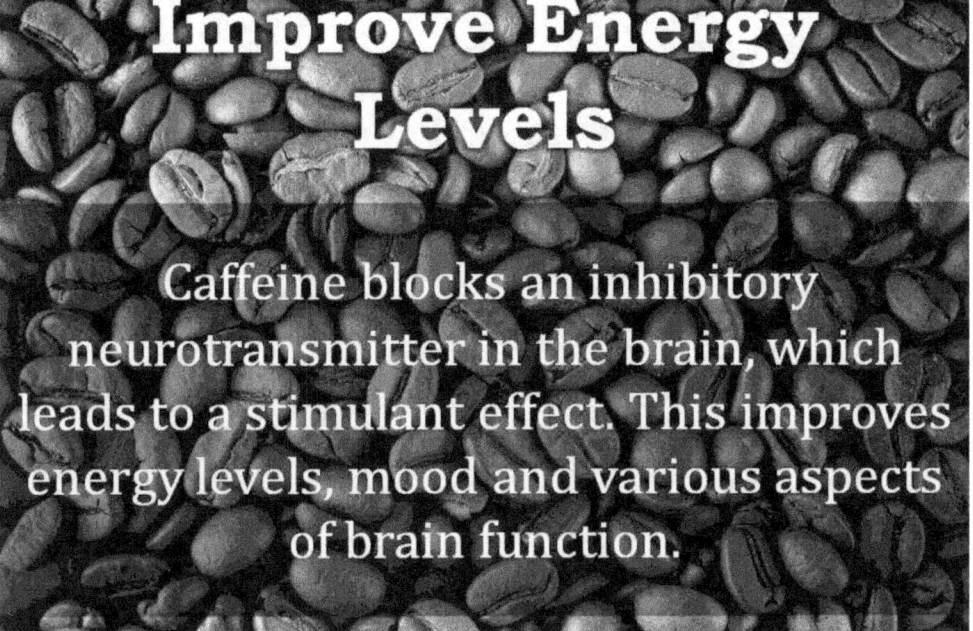

Improve Energy Levels

Caffeine blocks an inhibitory neurotransmitter in the brain, which leads to a stimulant effect. This improves energy levels, mood and various aspects of brain function.

51 SCIENTIFIC REASONS
COFFEE IS HEALTHY

01. Wakes you up
02. Improves your focus
03. Helps relieve headaches
04. Makes you smarter
05. Provides essential nutrients
06. A large source of antioxidants
07. Improves good cholesterol
08. Reduces inflammation
09. One of the lowest calorie drinks
10. Raises metabolic rate & burns fat
11. Keeps you hydrated
12. Improves physical performance
13. Preserves your muscles
14. Helps you workout harder
15. Reduces muscle soreness after exercise
16. Helps meet daily dietary fiber
17. Helps keep your bowel healthy
18. Lowers risk of colorectal cancer
19. Benefits gastrointestinal flora
20. Helps recover colon surgery quicker
21. Improves blood circulation
22. Enhances DNA repair
23. Protects against retinal damage
24. May protect against cataracts
25. Protects against eyelid spasm
26. Relieves symptoms of asthma
27. Lowers risk of gallstones
28. Lowers risk of kidney stones
29. Reduces risk of oral cancer
30. Lowers risk of liver cancer

31. Protects liver from cirrhosis
32. Lowers risk of prostate cancer
33. Lowers risk of endometrial cancer
34. Protects against estrogen receptor-negative breast cancer
35. Fights cardiovascular disease
36. Lowers risk of stroke in women
37. Great for your skin
38. Lowers stress
39. Fights depression
40. Lowers risk of Type II Diabetes
41. Protects against dementia
42. Lowers Alzheimer's disease
43. Lowers Parkinson's disease risk
44. Helps with your memory
45. Prevents ringing in the ears
46. Good for your teeth
47. Stimulates hair growth
48. Prevents erectile dysfunction
49. Perks up sperm
50. Protects against gout
51. May add years to your life!

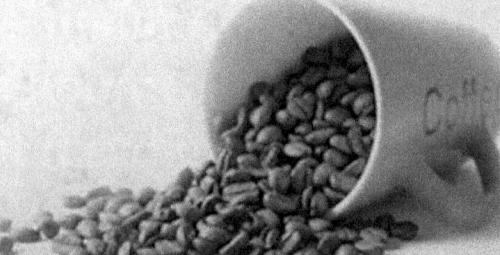

Coffee Is Actually Good For Health

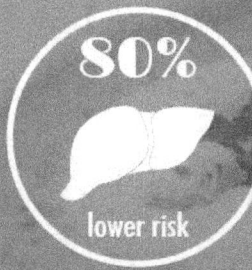

80%
lower risk

Protective Effects

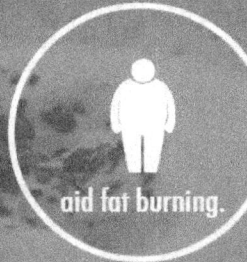

aid fat burning.

Help You Burn Fat

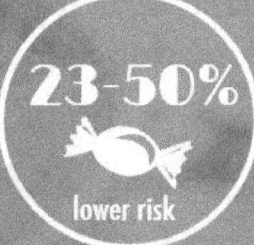

23-50%
lower risk

Lower Your Risk of Type II Diabetes

There Are Essential Nutrients in Coffee

40%

Studies show that coffee drinkers have up to a 40% lower risk of liver cancer.

Magnesium & Niacin
(Vitamin B3): 2% of the RDA

Pantothenic Acid
(Vitamin B5): 6% of the RDA.

Manganese & Potassium
3% of the RDA

Riboflavin
(Vitamin B2): 11% of the RDA

65%

Several studies show that coffee drinkers have up to a 65% lower risk of getting Alzheimer's disease.

For more information on health, nutrition, gardening, phytonutrition, antioxidants and loads more please visit my website and while you are there go ahead and subscribe to my phytonutrient blog – its free but the information is priceless!

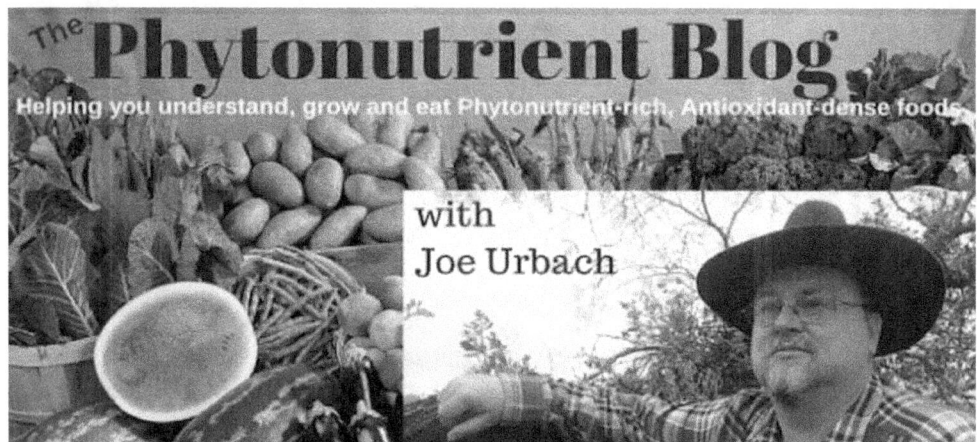

www.GardeningAustin.com/blog

For the highest quality, hand sourced, Organic, NON-GMO seeds for you garden visit:

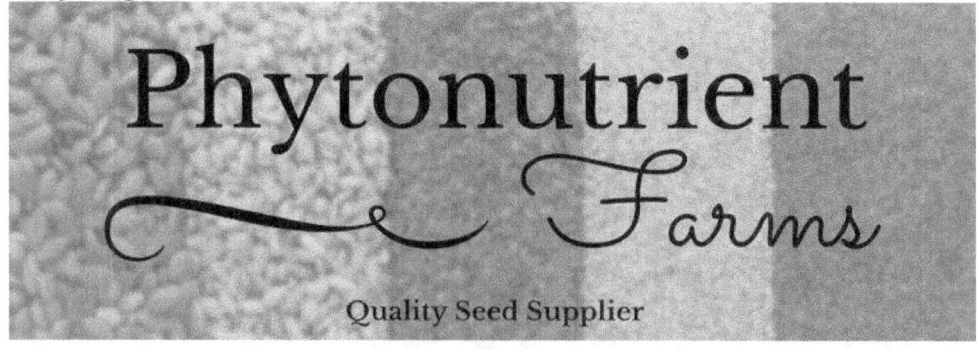

www.phytonutrientfarms.com

ANTIOXIDANT
PHYTONUTRIENTS

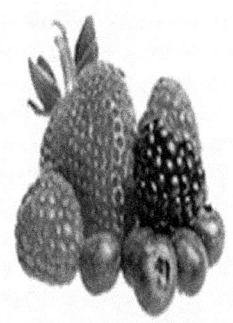

Many oxygen-radicals form during normal metabolism of nutrients. These oxygen-radicals (oxidants) are highly reactive and damage DNA molecules, proteins and cholesterol-rich LDL molecules.

Antioxidants include vitamins, minerals enzymes and phytonutrients.

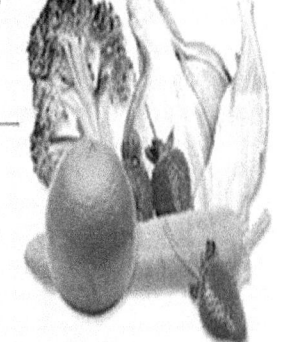

Phytonutrients protect us from a build-up of excess free radicals.

Tomatoes, broccoli, cauliflower and fruits of berry family are excellent sources of natural antioxidants.